THE
CARBOHYDRATE
ADDICT'S
COOKBOOK

250 All-New <u>Low-Carb</u> Recipes That Will Cut
Your Cravings and Keep You Slim for Life

Other Books by Drs. Richard and Rachael Heller

The Carbohydrate Addict's Calorie Counter
The Carbohydrate Addict's Carbohydrate Counter
The Carbohydrate Addict's Fat Counter
The Carbohydrate Addict's Gram Counter

The Carbohydrate Addict's Healthy Heart Program
The Carbohydrate Addict's LifeSpan Program
The Carbohydrate Addict's Diet
The Carbohydrate Addict's Healthy for Life Plan
The Carbohydrate Addict's Program for Success
Carbohydrate-Addicted Kids

Visit the Hellers' Website at:
www.carbohydrateaddicts.com

Dr. Richard F. Heller
Professor Emeritus, Mount Sinai School of Medicine
Professor Emeritus, Graduate Center of the City University of New York
Professor Emeritus, City University of New York

Dr. Rachael F. Heller
Assistant Professor Emeritus, Mount Sinai School of Medicine
Assistant Professor Emeritus, Graduate Center of the City University of New York

THE
CARBOHYDRATE
ADDICT'S
COOKBOOK

250 All-New <u>Low-Carb</u> Recipes That Will Cut
Your Cravings and Keep You Slim for Life

Dr. Richard F. Heller and
Dr. Rachael F. Heller

John Wiley & Sons, Inc.

New York   Chichester   Weinheim   Brisbane   Singapore   Toronto

Published by John Wiley & Sons, Inc.
Published simultaneously in Canada

Design and production by Navta Associates, Inc.

This publication is designed to provide accurate and authoritative information in regard to the subject matter covered. It is sold with the understanding that the publisher is not engaged in rendering professional services. If professional advice or other expert assistance is required, the services of a competent professional person should be sought.

ISBN: 0-471-38290-6

Printed in the United States of America

10 9 8 7 6 5 4 3 2 1

The information in this book reflects the authors' experiences and is not intended to replace medical advice or the details and guidelines provided by a full and approved eating program. It is not the intent of the authors to diagnose or prescribe. The intent is only to offer information to help you cooperate with your physician in your mutual quest for desirable health. Only your physician can determine whether or not any diet or eating program is appropriate for you. Before embarking on any diet or eating program, or before incorporating the recipes in this book, you should consult your physician. In addition to regular checkups and supervision, any questions or symptoms should be addressed to your physician. In the event you use any information contained or implied herein without your physician's approval, you are prescribing for yourself and the publisher and authors assume no responsibility.

As with any program, one size cannot fit all, and your program should be individualized in conjunction with your physician. It is important that together you develop your own specific program based on your physician's advice and your own particular requirements and preferences, so that you may derive the best benefit from this program. As in all matters, your physician's recommendations should be primary.

The recipes in this book are not intended for pregnant or nursing women or for children or teens or those with overt or covert medical conditions. Their needs are so specialized that they cannot be addressed here.

The authors are not responsible for unintentional errors, misprints, or changes that might have occurred in the production of this book.

Notice: The terms "Reward Meal," "Carbohydrate Addict's Diet," "Carbohydrate Addict," and derivatives and abbreviations are registered and service trademarks owned by Drs. Richard and Rachael Heller and cannot be used without their written permission.

To every dieter,
who deserves the right to enjoy, without guilt,
all of the pleasures that life has to offer.

Contents

Acknowledgments

We wish to express our deep appreciation to:

Mel Berger of the William Morris Agency, by far and away the best agent and advisor in the world. His thoughtful and incisive advice, common sense, creativity, years of experience, caring, and hard work make him the best agent and the best friend anyone could ever have.

Tom Miller, our remarkable editor, for his unswerving interest, commitment, creativity, and hard work in making this book the best it could be and making it available to all who need it.

Lisa Vaia, our associate managing editor, whose attention to detail, commitment, and expertise have eased the way for this book's authors and for all the readers yet to come.

Miriam V. Sarzin, our copyeditor, who worked hard and long (and very well!) to make this book a most user-friendly adventure in cooking.

Thanks to Karen Fraley, our proofreader, for her eagle eye and fine mind.

Donna Bagdasarian, Mel Berger's most capable assistant, whose trusted reliability, concern, and loving nature have proven precious and essential assets.

Deborah Nicolai, Jonathan Martin, and Caroline Jean (in order of appearance in this world), who bring joy and laughter to our lives.

Barbara Scherer, the Administrator of CASupport, for her love and devotion to helping those whose lives have been made better by all of her hard work and very long hours.

Ron Gordon, Ph.D., who gave us the helping hand we needed when we really needed it.

Norman Katz, who is valued by so many and with good reason.

Hal Ackerstein, M.D., whose intelligence and quick wit match his generosity of spirit.

Leslie St. Louis, M.D., for his integrity, wide range of knowledge, generous concern, and very wise counsel.

Douglas E. Hertford, M.D., for his interest, sincerity, and expert advice.

Martin W. Weber, who is always there when needed and whose interest and ability to ask the right questions at the right time, and to give the right answers as well, have proven invaluable and unerringly on target.

Margaret Boulineau and her superb staff at the Comfort Inn in Lake Buena Vista, Florida, for making us a wonderful home away from home on our frequent visits to Walt Disney World where we both work and play hard.

To Andy, Joseph, Jack, Scott, Mike, and Dave at Interwrx, our excellent Web host (at http://www.interwrx.com) who have worked day and night to help us stay on the net and do our job.

To Carl Page, Beth, Sergio, Allison, Jennifer, and Melissa and at www.egroups.com who have made it possible to keep CASupport a vital support network.

The Apple Computer Company and their support staff, for the development, care, and "feeding" of our user-friendly Powerbooks and PowerMacs that have made our lives wonderful. They have been invaluable tools in all of our work. It is all of Apple's hard work that has made work easy for us.

We've saved the "littlest" for last and that makes it all the sweeter: We wish to acknowledge Molly Berger, our young agent-in-training, confidant, cheerleader, and publicist-in-training par excellence.

INTRODUCTION
and
GREETINGS

Hello!

Welcome to *The Carbohydrate Addict's Cookbook!*

We're glad you found us!

We have developed each of the recipes in this book to bring you a wide variety of exciting, new, delicious, and easy low-carbohydrate meals.

Any of the recipes you find in this book can be included in low-carbohydrate meals* in all of the following:

The Carbohydrate Addict's LifeSpan Program

The Carbohydrate Addict's Diet

The Carbohydrate Addict's Healthy for Life Plan
   (formerly known as *Healthy for Life*)

Carbohydrate-Addicted Kids

The Carbohydrate Addict's Healthy Heart Program

These recipes can be enjoyed on all of the following as well:

   Atkins diets

   Protein Power programs

   The Zone programs

   Sugar Busters diets

   or any other low-carbohydrate eating program.

Important Note: Our programs are NOT low-carbohydrate diets. We do NOT ask you to restrict the amount of carbohydrate you take in each day.

On our programs, balanced carbohydrate-rich Reward Meals will provide your body with the carbohydrate-rich foods you need and love every day, while additional low-carbohydrate meals will help balance your blood insulin levels.

---

*Carbohydrate Addict's programs include both low-carbohydrate meals and a Reward Meal® each day. If you are following any of the Carbohydrate Addict's programs and include the recipes found in this book in your Reward Meals, be certain to balance with healthy, carbohydrate-rich grains, vegetables, fruits, and desserts as well. For all programs, follow your physician's recommendations.

A Very Simple Goal

For the carbohydrate addict, less insulin means fewer and far less intense carbohydrate cravings and a natural, struggle-free weight loss. Balanced insulin levels also lead to a reduction in the body's resistance to insulin, reducing virtually all of the insulin-related risk factors associated with high blood pressure, atherosclerosis, high blood fat levels, heart disease, and adult-onset diabetes.

Each of our books describes an insulin-balancing program that incorporates a single daily well-balanced carbohydrate-rich meal (usually called the Reward Meal) and other daily meals and snacks that are low in carbohydrates.

Any recipe you find in this book can, of course, be included in any Reward Meal as well as in low-carbohydrate meals.

So sit back and read on!

Options, Tips, Health-Smart Choices

All of the recipes that follow are nutritious, delicious, and—best of all—they are legal! So enjoy each of the low-carbohydrate dishes that follow while reducing or eliminating your carbohydrate cravings, losing weight, and living guilt-free!

In the pages that follow, feel free to mix, match, and combine the dishes you find in this book. The vegetable dishes and protein dishes are meant to complement each other and provide you with a whole new world of choices.

While the choice is yours, assuming that your physician agrees, whenever possible we recommend that you replace the saturated fats in your diet with olive oil. Unsaturated fats such as olive oil have been shown to be highly beneficial for health and are much preferred over the animal fats and trans fatty acids found in butter, margarines, and hydrogenated cooking oils.

For those concerned with the total fat content of a recipe, appropriate low-fat alternatives may be used, but be aware that some alternatives can contain added sugars or other carbohydrates and are therefore inappropriate substitutes.

Where mayonnaise is a listed ingredient, unless your physician indicates otherwise, we prefer the use of a "regular" mayonnaise. Do not substitute "low-fat" varieties for regular mayonnaise; low-fat varieties of mayonnaise often contain several forms of sugar to replace the fat that has been removed. Added sugars can mean higher levels of insulin that can lead to hunger, cravings, weight gain, and increased risk for heart disease and adult-onset diabetes.

If you wish, the fat content of a regular mayonnaise can be reduced by thinning it with a little water. By adding a little water at a time and mixing well, you can reduce the fat content of regular mayonnaise by one-fourth to one-third without adding any sugar. It is surprising how little effect the water has on the consistency of the mayonnaise.

We have included some recipes that dish up several servings. These dishes result in easy leftovers or provide extra meals for the family (when a carbohydrate balance is included for non-dieters). Should you prefer fewer (or a greater number of) servings, remember that recipes in this book can be adjusted. If, for example, a recipe states that it serves four, and only two servings are required, then divide all of the ingredients by two. Likewise, for parties and celebrations, you are free to multiply quantities of ingredients by two or three or more!

Microwave ovens can be a real blessing for those who encounter serious time constraints in their lives. Many of the recipes in this book that may be frozen or refrigerated after preparation can be easily and quickly enjoyed when reheated in a microwave oven.

The guidelines of our programs can be adapted to comply with the current recommendations of the U.S. Surgeon General's *Report on Nutrition and Health;* the U.S. Department of Agriculture and the Department of Health and Human Services' *Report on Dietary Guidelines for Americans,* and the American Heart Association's *Eating Plan for Healthy Americans.*

Here are some suggestions for incorporating these agencies' dietary guidelines:

Incorporating Low-Fat, Low-Saturated-Fat, Low-Salt, and Other Healthy Agency Dietary Recommendations* into Your Program

> Before incorporating any dietary guideline into your program, you should consult your physician. Only your doctor can determine which recommendations are appropriate to you and your individual health needs and how best to incorporate health agency recommendations.

Health Agency Recommendation #1

Eat a variety of foods.

To include recommendation #1 into your program:
Add new foods into your low-carbohydrate meals and choose from a variety of salad ingredients, low-carbohydrate vegetables, proteins, and low-carbohydrate dairy items. Try one new vegetable each week and enjoy the new recipes you find in the pages that follow. It's fun to explore an entirely new world of eating while continuing to enjoy your long-time favorites.

Health Agency Recommendation #2

Balance the food you eat with physical activity.
Maintain or improve your weight.

To include recommendation #2 into your program:
Many of our programs include activity options that can go a long way toward helping you make gradual changes that can lead to healthy, lifelong habits. As appropriate, start with small steps and, before making any changes, check with your physician.

---

*Adapted from the U.S. Surgeon General's *Report on Nutrition and Health;* the U.S. Department of Agriculture and the Department of Health and Human Services' *Report on Dietary Guidelines for Americans,* and the American Heart Association's *Eating Plan for Healthy Americans.*

Health Agency Recommendation #3

Choose a diet with plenty of grain products,
vegetables, and fruits.

To include recommendation #3 into your program:
In your low-carbohydrate meals, be sure to include a wide variety of fiber-rich low-carbohydrate vegetables.

Health Agency Recommendation #4

Choose a diet low in fat, saturated fat,
and cholesterol.

To include recommendation #4 into your program:
As part of a healthful eating plan, choose foods low in saturated fats. To reduce saturated fats, choose olive oil instead of heavy tropical or other saturated oils and avoid saturated fats (found in butter, other dairy, and meats), hydrogenated fats (saturated or unsaturated) and trans fatty acids (often found in margarine).

Health Agency Recommendation #5

Choose a diet moderate in sugars.

To include recommendation #5 into your program:
The basic guidelines of the Carbohydrate Addict's Programs and Plans will help you reduce your intake of sugar naturally.

By the very design of the program, your low-carbohydrate meals will essentially be sugar-free and, if at your Reward Meals you choose desserts made of complex carbohydrates like popcorn, pretzels, whole grain breads, or low-fat whole grain snacks rather than intensely sweet desserts, you can further help keep your intake of sugar low.

Health Agency Recommendation #6

Choose a diet moderate in salt (sodium).

To include recommendation #6 into your program:
At all meals, choose low-salt varieties of canned and packaged foods as well as low-salt cheese and other dairy products. Limit the amount of salt you add while cooking or at the table. When you are out at a restaurant, ask for low-salt alternatives and, when possible, avoid smoked and salted products.

Health Agency Recommendation #7

If you drink alcoholic beverages, do so in moderation.

To include recommendation #7 into your program:
When alcoholic beverages are consumed, they should be consumed only in moderation and only during high-carbohydrate Reward Meals. Reward Meal balancing will naturally help keep your intake of alcoholic beverages to a moderate level. Always consult your physician; diabetics and others may be advised by their physicians to refrain from all alcohol.

In Addition to the Agency Recommendations above, the American Heart Association Makes the Following Recommendations*:

Total fat intake should be no more 30 percent of total calories;
    Saturated fatty acid intake should be no more than 8 to 10 percent of total calories;
    Polyunsaturated fatty acid intake should be no more than 10 percent of total calories;
    Cholesterol intake should be less than 300 milligrams per day;

* The American Heart Association's *Eating Plan for Healthy Americans,* 1996.

Sodium intake should be less than 2,400 milligrams per day; which is about 1¼ teaspoons of sodium chloride (salt);

Carbohydrate intake should make up 55 to 60 percent or more of calories, with emphasis on increasing sources of complex carbohydrates;

Total calories should be adjusted to achieve and maintain a healthy body weight.

Incorporating the American Heart Association's Recommendations into the Carbohydrate Addict's Programs:

To help adapt your program to better comply with the American Heart Association's guidelines:

Select proteins that are lower in saturated fat. For example, choose tofu (soybean curd), soybean-based protein, and fish rather than fatty cuts of animal protein.

When eating prepared foods, choose low-salt varieties; at home, cook with very little salt.

In order to be sure of including the recommended proportion of carbohydrates, choose fowl, fish, and tofu as your proteins. These lower-calorie proteins in combination with low-carbohydrate vegetables will afford you the ability of maintaining the 55 to 60 percentage of carbohydrate calories without overloading the carbohydrate balance of your high-carbohydrate Reward Meal.

If, in addition, you consume mostly high-quality complex carbohydrates, you can comply with the American Heart Association's recommendation to keep calories low and to maintain an emphasis on complex carbohydrates while keeping sugar intake low.

First Things First

Although the recipes in this book can be adapted to almost any carbohydrate-regulating eating plan, we urge you to select a program such as ours, which encourages you to eat, every day, the carbohydrates you need and love, and that are essential to your health. Remember, you don't have to give up carbohydrates in order to lose your cravings and your weight.

Since all of the recipes in this book are low in carbohydrates and high in fiber and protein, they should NOT make up your entire eating program. These foods are meant to be consumed in combination with other balancing foods every day.*

Just one final note: It is important to remember that only the patient and physician in consultation can determine which health agency dietary guidelines are appropriate, and how best to incorporate them into an eating plan. We therefore strongly advise you to consult with your physician before you make any changes in your eating. After all, to borrow a phrase, you're worth it!

*For details, see our books on carbohydrate addiction, listed in the front of this book.

APPETIZERS
and
SOUPS

If we had our own way, our entire meal would consist of nothing but appetizers. Sometimes, we do just that. Add a nice warm soup in winter or a cold soup and salad in summer, and we are two very happy people.

Come join us as we share with you some of our favorite low-carb treats.

Marinated Thai Chicken

By their very nature, many Thai dishes offer great low-carb choices. We like to skewer the cooked chicken chunks on toothpicks, along with green pepper chunks, and serve alongside cool cucumber slices.

3 tablespoons olive oil	1 teaspoon ground cumin
1 tablespoon teriyaki sauce*	1 small dried hot pepper, finely crumbled
3 cloves garlic, minced	salt to taste
1 tablespoon grated fresh ginger	ground black pepper to taste
1 tablespoon curry powder	2 pounds boneless, skinless chicken breasts
1 teaspoon ground coriander	
1 teaspoon ground turmeric	

In a large bowl, combine olive oil, teriyaki sauce, garlic, ginger, curry, coriander, turmeric, cumin, hot pepper, salt, and black pepper.

Cut the chicken into bite-size chunks. Place in marinade, cover, and refrigerate overnight.

Just prior to serving, preheat the oven to 450°F.

Remove chicken chunks from marinade and discard marinade.

Place chicken chunks on an aluminum foil–lined baking sheet and bake for 4 to 6 minutes.

---

*Most recent Carbohydrate Addict's books may contain alternative guidelines for this ingredient. Consult your book's food lists for guidance. Use acceptable alternative as appropriate.

Spiced Olives

Rachael's neighbor and baby-sitter, Angela, prepared meals that made you feel good all over. Angela's table was the only place where there were no disapproving looks and restrictions. Though olives are supposed to be an "adult" food, Rachael loved these then as she does now.

20 large olives, rinsed and drained

1 tablespoon orange zest, finely grated

3 tablespoons extra virgin olive oil

2 cloves garlic, minced

$\frac{1}{2}$ teaspoon dried thyme

$\frac{1}{8}$ teaspoon ground allspice

$\frac{1}{4}$ teaspoon coarse salt

$\frac{1}{4}$ teaspoon coarsely ground pepper

1 tablespoon fresh parsley, chopped

Rinse the olives in cold water, then drain well. Place the olives, orange zest, oil, and garlic in a bowl and mix well.

Add the thyme, allspice, salt, and pepper. Combine well.

Add the parsley. Pack the olives into an airtight container and refrigerate, covered, for 2 to 3 days for the flavors to meld.

Tangy Shrimp

We think that the best-kept dining secret at Disney World is Chef Mickey's buffet in the Contemporary Hotel. While the monorail rides above you, and the characters cavort around you, you can enjoy all the succulent shrimp (and other foods) you desire. This shrimp dish is inspired by that memorable eating experience.

1 pound raw jumbo bay shrimp	1 tablespoon fresh thyme, chopped
2 tablespoons olive oil	½ teaspoon ground black pepper
1 tablespoon garlic, minced	cayenne pepper to taste
1 tablespoon fresh rosemary, chopped	¼ teaspoon salt
	1 lemon, quartered

Peel and devein the shrimp, leaving the tails intact.

Combine the shrimp with the olive oil, garlic, rosemary, thyme, black pepper, cayenne pepper, and salt.

Marinate in refrigerator for 1 hour.

Lay the shrimp in a dry nonstick skillet over medium-high heat. Cook, turning once, for 4 to 8 minutes, depending on shrimp size. Brush the shrimp with the remaining marinade before turning.

Serve with lemon quarters.

Cheddar Cheese Dip

When friends, family, and readers want a tip on how to get themselves to eat more low-carb veggies, we give them this recipe and smile, knowing that they are about to enjoy a special treat that will make their low-carb meals a delight.

2	tablespoons olive oil	1	egg, beaten*
1	pound sharp Cheddar cheese, shredded	1	teaspoon dry mustard
		1	teaspoon paprika
1	cup sour cream		

Place olive oil in top of double boiler and add cheese.

Place over simmering water and stir until cheese begins to melt.

Add sour cream gradually, stirring constantly until cheese is melted and mixture is smooth.

Stir in egg, mustard, and paprika.

Serve at once while still warm with celery, green peppers, mushrooms, cucumbers, or raw or lightly steamed green beans or cauliflower.

*Use certified, salmonella-free eggs only.

Swedish Meatballs

On a rainy, cold winter weekend, we love to settle ourselves in with a good video while enjoying these meatballs and some low-carb veggies and dip.

1 pound ground beef	1 large egg, lightly beaten
1 small onion, finely grated	salt to taste
1 tablespoon finely chopped garlic	ground black pepper to taste
1 teaspoon ground allspice	2 tablespoons olive oil
1/4 teaspoon ground nutmeg	1/4 cup water
1/4 cup chopped fresh dill	1 tablespoon white wine

In a large bowl, combine the beef, onion, garlic, allspice, nutmeg, dill, egg, salt, and pepper.

Form into 30 meatballs, about 1 inch in diameter.

Put olive oil in a large nonstick skillet and heat over medium heat.

Place half of the meatballs in the skillet and cook, shaking the skillet occasionally, until meatballs are browned on all sides and cooked through, 8 to 10 minutes. Remove to a paper towel to drain.

Repeat for second half of meatballs.

Pour off the residual oil in the skillet and add the water and wine.

Cook over high heat, scraping up any browned bits on the bottom, until the liquid is somewhat reduced, about 4 minutes.

Add the meatballs back to the pan and cook for 10 minutes, spooning the sauce over the meatballs as it thickens.

Serve immediately.

Hard-Boiled Eggs Italiano

The subtle blend of flavors provided by the cheeses and garlic makes this a special treat!

½ cup dried basil	⅔ cup olive oil
1 large clove garlic, minced	salt to taste
1½ tablespoons grated Parmesan cheese	black pepper to taste
1 tablespoon grated Romano cheese	8 hard-boiled eggs, shelled

In a food processor, prepare a pesto sauce by combining basil, garlic, Parmesan cheese, and Romano cheese.

While continuing to blend, add olive oil in a slow, steady stream.

Season with salt and pepper.

Place in an appropriate container and refrigerate overnight.

When ready to serve, cut eggs into wedges and arrange on a bed of lettuce or fresh spinach on a serving platter.

Drizzle pesto over eggs and serve.

Chicken Liver Pâté

It's still amazing to us that we can enjoy an elegant pâté like this and still be watching our carbs. Richard loves this recipe spread on green pepper slices or rolled in lettuce leaves. For canapés, we put dollops of it on cucumber slices (with peel intact).

3–4 tablespoons olive oil	pinch cayenne pepper
1 clove garlic, minced	½ teaspoon ground nutmeg
¼ cup diced celery	¼ teaspoon ground cloves
1 pound chicken livers	2 tablespoons teriyaki
½ teaspoon salt	sauce*

Put 3 tablespoons olive oil in a skillet over a medium heat. Sauté garlic and celery until just soft.

Add livers and cook until done. Discard the liquid and cool the livers.

Place in a blender or food processor, add liver and all remaining ingredients, and purée until well combined. Add another tablespoon olive oil as needed.

Pack into 1½-pint bowl and chill thoroughly.

*Most recent Carbohydrate Addict's books may contain alternative guidelines for this ingredient. Consult your book's food lists for guidance. Use acceptable alternative as appropriate.

Parmesan Oysters

There's a breakfast buffet in Sarasota, Florida, where you overlook the lake while you eat. They serve the best oysters that we have ever eaten. The first time we sampled the recipe that inspired these oysters, we saw an alligator silently sail by in the lake below. We could hardly believe our eyes—or our taste buds—that day.

2 dozen whole oysters

1 clove garlic, minced

1 tablespoon minced fresh parsley

2 teaspoons teriyaki sauce*

2 tablespoons clam juice

1/2 cup olive oil

2 tablespoons grated Parmesan cheese

1/2 cup finely chopped mushrooms

salt to taste

ground black pepper to taste

Preheat oven to 400°F.

Shuck oysters, drain, and reserve half the shells.

Combine garlic, parsley, teriyaki sauce, and clam juice with 6 tablespoons olive oil.

Dip each oyster into sauce and place in a shell on a baking pan. Spoon remaining sauce over oysters.

Sprinkle cheese and a teaspoon of chopped mushrooms on each oyster. Dribble with remaining 2 tablespoons olive oil.

Bake for 15 minutes.

*Most recent Carbohydrate Addict's books may contain alternative guidelines for this ingredient. Consult your book's food lists for guidance. Use acceptable alternative as appropriate.

Seafood Starter

We especially enjoy this dish when we serve it as a low-carb dinner. Elegant and sophisticated, it's especially good with Spiced Olives (page 13).

6 ounces flounder fillet	1 teaspoon dry white wine
12 to 16 large sea scallops	2 tablespoons chopped fresh parsley
12 to 16 whole jumbo shrimp	2 tablespoons olive oil

Preheat oven to 400°F.

Cut flounder into 6 to 8 slices and place each slice in an oiled shell-shaped baking dish.

Arrange scallops and shrimp around flounder, pour wine over fish. Sprinkle with chopped parsley and oil.

Bake until fish is flaky and thoroughly cooked.

Mushrooms Allegro

Traveling through the Florida Keys, we stumbled on a most wonderful restaurant. Its owners were brilliant chefs, every dish was exquisite, and many inspired us to develop our own variations, such as this one. We don't go to the Keys much any more, but it's almost worth the trip just for the eating.

1 pound mushrooms	2 tablespoons white vinegar
½ cup water	1 tablespoon salt
2 tablespoons olive oil	dash dried basil
½ clove garlic, chopped	2 bay leaves
dash peppercorns	2 tablespoons fresh lemon juice
dash ground thyme	

Slice mushrooms in half through stems. Put in a bowl and set aside.

Combine remaining ingredients in a medium saucepan and heat but do not boil.

Pour sauce over mushrooms. Refrigerate overnight. Remove peppercorns and bay leaves before serving.

Buttery Escargots

Bet you can't eat just a half dozen! We love these on top of steamed or sautéed spinach.

1 stick butter	3 ounces chicken stock, homemade only (page 26), or water
2 tablespoons olive oil	
8 cloves garlic, chopped fine	¼ cup dry Madeira wine
48 large snails, with shells	½ teaspoon salt
2 tablespoons chopped fresh parsley	

Preheat oven to 425°F.

Place butter in saucepan and cook until it begins to turn brown. Do not burn.

Add olive oil and garlic and sauté until light brown.

Remove snails from shells, leaving shells intact.

Add snails and sauté for approximately 1 minute.

Add parsley, chicken stock (or water), Madeira, and salt. Cook until liquid is reduced to about one-quarter.

Place a little of the sauce in each shell, then add a snail. Reserve the remaining sauce.

Place snails in shells in a baking dish and heat in oven for approximately 2 minutes. Pour reserved sauce over snails and serve.

Holiday Meatball Appetizer

SERVES 8

We make the entire recipe for just the two of us and enjoy this dish over the course of several meals. We add tomato sauce for Reward Meals and vary the low-carb veggies. We crumble meatballs up and add them to salads, too!

2 pounds lean ground beef

1 cup minced celery

2 eggs, beaten

2 tablespoons teriyaki sauce*

3 cloves garlic, finely chopped

½ teaspoon salt

black pepper to taste

Place ground beef, celery, eggs, teriyaki sauce, garlic, salt, and pepper in a large bowl.

Form into meatballs about ¾ inch in diameter.

Place the meatballs in a large nonstick skillet over medium heat, and brown all around.

When cooked through, place on a platter with a supply of toothpicks and serve immediately.

*Most recent Carbohydrate Addict's books may contain alternative guidelines for this ingredient. Consult your book's food lists for guidance. Use acceptable alternative as appropriate.

Herbed Cheese Dip

SERVES 12

*We love the smooth and creamy texture of this dish and the
special flavor that all the herbs bring.*

8 ounces Cheddar cheese, crumbled	1 tablespoon dried parsley
	¼ teaspoon dried thyme
1 clove garlic	¼ teaspoon dried dill weed
1 tablespoon fresh chives, cut in 3-inch pieces	
	8 ounces cream cheese
1 tablespoon dried basil	2 tablespoons sour cream

Place Cheddar cheese into bowl of food processor with
chopping blade intact.

Mash garlic clove with flat edge of knife or in garlic
press and add to processor bowl.

Add chives, basil, parsley, thyme, and dill. Add more
additional spices or herbs as you desire. Process just until
herbs are chopped.

Add cream cheese and sour cream.

Process until desired consistency, adding more sour
cream for a softer spread. Makes about one pint.

Peppered Seafood Appetizer

SERVES 8

The only problem with this appetizer is that you might want to keep eating it for the entire low-carb meal. But then again, you're allowed to do just that!

1/4 cup olive oil	1/2 teaspoon minced dried hot chile
1/4 cup fresh lemon juice, strained for seeds	1/8 teaspoon dried thyme
3 teaspoons minced fresh dill weed	1 teaspoon paprika
3 cloves garlic, minced	1/4 teaspoon ground black pepper
2 bay leaves, crushed	1 1/2 pounds flounder fillets

In a large bowl, whisk together olive oil, 1/4 cup lemon juice, dill weed, garlic, bay leaves, hot chile, thyme, paprika, and black pepper.

Add the fish and turn in the marinade to make sure that all sides are covered. Refrigerate for at least 2 hours before cooking.

When ready to cook, place a large skillet over a medium heat, add fish with marinade. Cook lightly but thoroughly.

Serve warm.

Basic Chicken Stock

We make this stock in great quantities, then freeze it in small plastic freezer bags to be used for several weeks to come. A wonderful low-carbohydrate comfort food, it's good for the healing of colds and the reduction of stressful days.

1	whole chicken carcass	1	bay leaf
2	quarts water	¼	teaspoon dried basil
1	celery stalk	6	whole peppercorns
1	small onion, quartered	¼	cup chopped fresh parsley

Break up carcass. Add giblets and/or extra chicken (raw or cooked) if available and desired.

Combine all ingredients in a large soup kettle.

Bring to a boil and simmer, uncovered, over low heat for 1½ to 2 hours.

Cool the broth, strain, and discard solids. Freeze in small zip-top bags for future use.

Variations: Use ½ pound of fish fillets or beef roast (with beef bones, if available) for a tasty fish or beef stock.

Aromatic Shrimp Soup

It's difficult to find a low-carbohydrate soup that tastes good, but we've found that this one is a happy exception.

2 tablespoons olive oil	¹/₂ teaspoon dried thyme
2 large cloves garlic, minced	6 cups chicken stock, homemade only (page 26), or water
4 celery stalks, diced	
2 medium green bell peppers, diced	1¹/₂ pounds jumbo shrimp, peeled and deveined
6 tablespoons mayonnaise	
¹/₂ teaspoon paprika	black pepper to taste
¹/₂ teaspoon dried oregano	¹/₄ cup minced fresh parsley

Heat olive oil in a large saucepan over medium heat.

Add garlic, celery, and green pepper and sauté until vegetables soften, about 5 minutes.

Add mayonnaise, paprika, oregano, and thyme and sauté until fragrant, about 1 minute.

Add chicken stock (or water) and bring to boil.

Cook over medium-high heat about 30 minutes, or until thickened.

Add shrimp and simmer about 4 minutes, or until shrimp are opaque and cooked through. Season with black pepper.

Ladle a portion of shrimp into each warm soup plate, sprinkle with parsley, and serve immediately.

Chilled Cauliflower Soup

We love cold soups in the summer. When we add protein and salad, it's hard to believe that this makes a low-carbohydrate meal. By the way, we especially enjoy a sprig of mint in the middle of the bowl for looks and taste.

1 head cauliflower, chopped	1 tablespoon dry sherry
½ teaspoon fresh lemon juice	1 cup heavy cream
	salt to taste
2 cups chicken stock, homemade only (page 26), or water	cayenne pepper to taste
	dried basil to taste

Purée cauliflower in a blender with lemon juice.

Blend in chicken stock and sherry.

Pour into a bowl and whisk in cream. Season to taste with salt, cayenne, and basil.

Chill.

BREAKFASTS

Breakfasts are not just for the start of the day anymore. As snacks or treats, brunch or lunch, we enjoy breakfasts anytime.

Our favorite weekend breakfasts entail sleeping late (or at least until 9:00 A.M.), watching a bit of early TV or the last bit of a video that we fell asleep on the night before, a leisurely shower or bath (even better), and an unhurried brunch.

Ahhh, feels good just thinking of it!

Warm and Wonderful Baked Brie

A good friend of ours introduced us to this simple preparation. Once spoiled, we could never eat plain old cold Brie again. We usually split a wheel between us and scoop up the warm, luscious cheese with cucumber coins or mushroom caps. It's so good!

1 small wheel Brie,
   quartered

Preheat oven to 350°F.

Place the four pieces of Brie on an ovenproof serving platter with a 1-inch-deep rim.

Bake until softened and slightly runny, 18 to 20 minutes.

Baked Buffalo Wings

Store-bought wings can be full of preservatives and additives, so we invented this recipe for on-the-go breakfasts that we know we can trust.

3	tablespoons olive oil	6	ounces Roquefort cheese
¼	cup Tabasco or other hot pepper sauce	1	cup sour cream
2	tablespoons white vinegar	2	tablespoons mayonnaise
20	chicken wing drumettes		ground pepper to taste
	paprika to taste	4	large celery stalks, cut into sticks

Preheat oven to 350°F.

Lightly coat a baking sheet with 1 tablespoon of olive oil.

Mix remaining 2 tablespoons olive oil with hot pepper sauce and vinegar.

Dip chicken into mixture and arrange on baking sheet. Sprinkle lightly with paprika.

Bake until crisp and brown, about 30 minutes.

While chicken drumettes are baking, prepare dip. Place Roquefort, sour cream, and mayonnaise in a medium bowl and mix together until smooth.

Season dip with pepper and serve with wings and celery sticks.

Broiled Sausage with Mustard

For us, mustard is a staple, like salt and pepper. Adding it to foods while they cook is something most most people have not tried. Once you experience it, we think you'll understand why we enjoy it so much.

4 medium Italian sausage links or patties	4 tablespoons Dijon mustard

Preheat broiler.

Place sausage pieces on a baking tray lined with aluminum foil. Top each link or patty with mustard and broil for 5 minutes, turning once and reapplying mustard during the broiling.

Dijon Creme in Salmon Rolls

One of the most elegant hotels in New York serves this every Sunday for brunch. We've improved on their recipe, we think, and we serve it without fancy chandeliers or a $100 breakfast bill!

¹/₂ cup mayonnaise	dash teriyaki sauce*
1¹/₂ tablespoons Dijon mustard	¹/₃ cup heavy cream
dash lemon juice	8 large slices smoked salmon

In a medium bowl combine and blend together mayonnaise, mustard, lemon juice, and teriyaki sauce.

Whip cream until soft peaks form and fold into mayonnaise mixture.

Lay salmon slices flat and cut in half crosswise. Place a small portion of mayonnaise mixture on each half slice.

Roll up the salmon and place on a dish lined with a lettuce leaf. Repeat the process until all smoked salmon slices have been filled.

*Most recent Carbohydrate Addict's books may contain alternative guidelines for this ingredient. Consult your book's food lists for guidance. Use acceptable alternative as appropriate.

Cheesy Horseradish Sticks

SERVES 4

We used to pack these up for breakfast several times a week and bring them to the office at Mount Sinai Hospital in New York. With the two of us crunching away, no one could get any work done until we had finished our morning ritual. They're especially good with a nice cup of coffee or tea.

½ pound Cheddar cheese, grated

4 ounces cream cheese

2 tablespoons mayonnaise

2 tablespoons prepared white horseradish

1 tablespoon minced garlic

½ teaspoon dry mustard

1 teaspoon teriyaki sauce*

dash salt

12 celery stalks, rinsed and dried

In a medium bowl, combine all the ingredients except celery, and blend until smooth.

Fill hollows of celery stalks with the mixture.

*Most recent Carbohydrate Addict's books may contain alternative guidelines for this ingredient. Consult your book's food lists for guidance. Use acceptable alternative as appropriate.

Canadian Bacon, Roasted Peppers, and Cheese

SERVES 2 TO 4

This is one of our Sunday morning favorites. We could probably have it more often, but we love to keep it as a treat for the weekends.

4 slices Canadian bacon*
1 teaspoon Dijon mustard
½ cup James's Roasted Capsicums, cut into strips (page 213)

⅛ teaspoon freshly ground black pepper
4 ounces Swiss cheese, sliced

Preheat broiler.

Line an oven pan with aluminum foil and place the slices of Canadian bacon on the foil.

Spread ¼ teaspoon mustard on each slice of Canadian bacon and cover with ⅛ cup green pepper strips. Season with freshly ground black pepper.

Add a slice of cheese to each. Broil for 3 to 4 minutes. Serve immediately.

*Most recent Carbohydrate Addict's books may contain alternative guidelines for this ingredient. Consult your book's food lists for guidance. Use acceptable alternative as appropriate.

Savory Spinach Omelet

Richard discovered this dish in the south of France. After the guests had arrived, the owner of the hotel simply left the premises for the weekend. She left a variation of this recipe and several pass keys tacked up on the refrigerator door. What fun!

2 large green bell peppers

½ cup spinach, washed and stemmed, or frozen equivalent, thawed and drained

dash salt

pinch freshly ground black pepper

dash grated nutmeg

1 tablespoon olive oil

4 eggs, beaten

½ teaspoon teriyaki sauce*

Wash peppers, remove tops and bottoms and discard the cores and seeds. Cut the peppers in half lengthwise.

Steam the pepper halves in a steamer (or in a covered pan in an inch of water) over medium-high heat for 18 to 20 minutes.

Remove the peppers from the pan and, when they are cool enough to handle, pull off the loose skin and cut into strips.

(continued on next page)

*Most recent Carbohydrate Addict's books may contain alternative guidelines for this ingredient. Consult your book's food lists for guidance. Use acceptable alternative as appropriate.

If using fresh spinach, place the leaves in the steamer and sprinkle with the salt, pepper, and nutmeg. Steam over medium-high heat for 1 to 2 minutes. Remove the spinach from the steamer and press out the juice with a fork. (If using frozen, drain and add salt, pepper, and nutmeg.)

Preheat a medium skillet over medium-low heat and wipe the bottom lightly with olive oil.

Pour the eggs into the pan. When the eggs are beginning to set, lay half the pieces of pepper across the middle of the pan. When the egg is set, flip the omelette and cook for 1 or 2 more minutes. Set aside and keep warm.

Place half the remaining green peppers and the teriyaki sauce into a blender and blend until smooth. Press the contents through a strainer into a bowl.

Cut the omelette into two equal parts and place on plates. Garnish with spinach and pepper sauce.

Saucy Cheese and Eggs

Block Island lies twelve miles off the coast of Rhode Island and our little pre–Civil War farmhouse there was our first home. Though the winter blasts could sometimes make drafts of cold air sweep through the rooms, we felt warm and happy when we started the day with this meal.

1 tablespoon olive oil	⅓ cup minced green bell peppers
8 eggs	2 tablespoons sliced black olives
1 teaspoon teriyaki sauce*	2 tablespoons chopped green chiles
1 teaspoon baking powder	sour cream for garnish (optional)
¼ teaspoon salt	
3 cups shredded Monterey Jack cheese	
1½ cups shredded Cheddar cheese	

Preheat oven to 375°F.

Oil a 9-inch square pan. Combine eggs and teriyaki sauce in a mixing bowl and beat until light and fluffy, about 5 minutes.

Add baking powder and salt. Mix well, then stir in cheeses, green pepper, olives, and green chiles.

Pour mixture into prepared pan and bake 20 to 25 minutes.

Let stand 5 minutes before serving. Cut into 8 pieces and serve.

Garnish with a dollop of sour cream, if desired.

*Most recent Carbohydrate Addict's books may contain alternative guidelines for this ingredient. Consult your book's food lists for guidance. Use acceptable alternative as appropriate.

Cold Chicken Roll-Up

When it's time to travel, we prepare these the night before, add some deviled eggs, and grab this breakfast as we rush out the door.

2 leftover baked chicken breasts

8 large lettuce leaves
   Dijon mustard

Slice the chicken breasts into lengthwise strips.

Place a thin coat of mustard on each lettuce leaf, layer in several strips of chicken, roll up the lettuce leaf.

Serve cold.

Hard-Boiled Delight

We should name this after our friend Ron, because it has a heart of gold.

4 tablespoons olive oil	2 tablespoons chopped fresh parsley
1 green bell pepper, seeded and chopped	
1 celery stalk, chopped	8 hard-boiled eggs, cooled and shelled
1 clove garlic, minced	¼ cup grated Parmesan cheese
6 ounces mushrooms, sliced	

Preheat oven to 375°F.

Place 2 tablespoons olive oil in a saucepan over medium heat and sauté pepper, celery, and garlic for 5 minutes.

Add mushrooms and sauté 5 more minutes. Add remaining 2 tablespoons olive oil and bring to a boil, stirring constantly.

Add parsley and sautéed vegetables to complete the sauce.

Slice eggs lengthwise. Spread a few tablespoons of the sauce over the bottom of an oiled casserole, top with some of the hard-boiled egg slices and sprinkle with sauce. Continue to make alternate layers of sauce and egg slices. End with a layer of sauce. Sprinkle thickly with grated Parmesan cheese.

Bake 20 minutes and serve warm.

Alpine Eggs

If you remain open to adventure, the world can offer some wonderful surprises! At a bus stop in Australia, we met a charming Swiss couple who offered this recipe to us in exchange for one of ours.

1 tablespoon olive oil	$1/2$ teaspoon black pepper
4 ounces Swiss cheese, sliced thin	$1/4$ cup heavy cream
4 eggs	$1/2$ cup grated Parmesan cheese
1 teaspoon salt	

Preheat oven to 350°F.

Coat the bottom of a shallow casserole dish with olive oil.

Line dish with thin cheese slices. Break the eggs neatly into the casserole dish, keeping them whole.

Add salt and pepper to cream, and carefully pour over the eggs.

Sprinkle with Parmesan cheese and bake for 10 minutes.

Brown the cheese topping under the broiler for 2 to 3 minutes, if necessary.

All-American Breakfast Ham Treat

SERVES 4

When Richard's youngest daughters were little, Richard used to make this dish for them. They thought it was something exotic and special and, much to their delight, he'd make up a new foreign-sounding name for it every time he served it.

1 cup chopped cooked ham	1 tablespoon Dijon mustard
1 cup diced celery	3 tablespoons mayonnaise
1 cup diced cauliflower	

Place all ingredients in large mixing bowl and toss until well coated.

Creamy Baked Eggs

SERVES 2 TO 4

If one of us has a cold, this has become our tried-and-true low-carbohydrate comfort food.

1 tablespoon olive oil	black pepper to taste
4 whole eggs	$\frac{1}{4}$ cup light cream
salt to taste	grated Parmesan cheese

Preheat oven to 350°F.
  Oil four custard cups.
  Break an egg carefully into each cup.
  Season with salt and pepper to taste.
  Pour 1 tablespoon of cream over each egg.
  Bake for 10 minutes.
  Sprinkle baked eggs with Parmesan cheese.

Salmon Rolls with Cream Cheese

Rachael loves to wrap these in large lettuce leaves and grab them when she's on the go. She likes them because they are simple and quick to make the night before and a nice change of pace for breakfast.

4 ounces cream cheese	½ teaspoon black pepper
1 tablespoon lemon juice	¼ pound smoked salmon,
1 tablespoon capers	thinly sliced

In a medium bowl, combine cream cheese, lemon juice, capers, and black pepper.

Spread on salmon slices and roll up. Chill and cut into bite-size pieces.

Broccoli and Eggs

This is a standard in our house, topped with cheese and with any leftover proteins thrown in for good measure. For this dish, we sometimes use spinach instead of broccoli.

2 tablespoons olive oil	4 hard-boiled eggs, shelled
1 teaspoon sesame oil	
3 tablespoons teriyaki sauce*	1 cup chopped broccoli*

Place olive oil, sesame oil, and teriyaki sauce in a skillet over medium heat. Mix with fork to distribute teriyaki sauce. Add eggs and cook gently for 5 minutes, basting and turning all the time until the eggs become dark brown.

Remove eggs to plate.

Quickly add broccoli and stir-fry until cooked but still crisp, approximately 3 minutes. Serve with eggs.

*Most recent Carbohydrate Addict's books may contain alternative guidelines for this ingredient. Consult your book's food lists for guidance. Use acceptable alternative as appropriate.

Breakfast Delhi Delight

*We discovered this easy-to-make dish in a little Indian grocery.
The cashier was eating it and it smelled great! Later, she invited
us to her home for some real home-style Indian cooking and we
discovered a new recipe and a new friend.*

¹/₂ cup mayonnaise	2 cups chopped cooked chicken
1 teaspoon fresh lemon juice	¹/₂ cup diced celery
2 tablespoons curry powder	¹/₂ cup diced green beans
	¹/₂ cup diced cauliflower

Blend mayonnaise, lemon juice, and curry powder until
smooth. Set aside.

Place remaining ingredients in a large bowl. Add mayonnaise sauce and toss well.

For best taste, let flavors blend in refrigerator for at
least 1 hour before serving.

Curried Eggs

We invented this dish one morning when we awakened with a craving for something simple but different. It's especially good wrapped in lettuce leaves. We'll bet you like it, too!

¹/₂ teaspoon finely chopped garlic	¹/₂ teaspoon curry powder
3 tablespoons olive oil	4 eggs

Sauté garlic in olive oil until soft, about 10 minutes.

Add curry powder and stir well.

Beat eggs slightly. Stir into the garlic mixture and cook over low heat, stirring occasionally until eggs are set.

Green Eggs without Ham

We missed poached eggs (they seem to have gone out of style, like succotash), so we updated them with some new tastes and textures. For a brunch or lunch, we particularly like these with cool cucumber slices and Canadian bacon.

1 package frozen chopped spinach	1 teaspoon dried basil
¼ cup olive oil	8 poached eggs
¼ cup heavy cream	¼ cup grated Parmesan cheese
1 teaspoon garlic, minced	

Preheat broiler.

Steam the spinach according to package directions. Drain thoroughly, squeezing out as much moisture as possible.

In a skillet over medium heat, combine 2 tablespoons olive oil, cream, garlic, and basil.

Coat the bottom of a baking dish with the remaining 2 tablespoons olive oil. Evenly layer the spinach in the dish.

Top spinach with the poached eggs. Pour cream sauce over all and sprinkle with cheese.

Broil for 5 to 10 minutes, or until top is brown.

Sandi's Chicken Salad

SERVES 2

Rachael's good friend Sandi always kept this in the refrigerator for a quick and tasty low-carb treat. Once we start to eat it, we get hooked on it for weeks at a time and enjoy it at meal after meal. Then we forget about it for a while, only to "rediscover" it and enjoy it all over again. This dish is also great with scallions and cheese and rolled up in romaine lettuce leaves.

½ tablespoon olive oil	1 teaspoon Dijon mustard
1 whole boneless, skinless chicken breast	juice of 1 lemon
2 tablespoons mayonnaise	2 celery stalks
1 tablespoon teriyaki sauce*	½ cup bean sprouts

Place oil in a small skillet and cook chicken over medium heat until thoroughly done on both sides, about 6 or 7 minutes per side.

While chicken is cooking, combine mayonnaise, teriyaki sauce, mustard, and lemon juice in a small bowl.

Chop celery into small pieces.

Drain chicken, cut into bite-size chunks, and mix with dressing in bowl.

Add chopped celery and sprouts.

*Most recent Carbohydrate Addict's books may contain alternative guidelines for this ingredient. Consult your book's food lists for guidance. Use acceptable alternative as appropriate.

Hearty Breakfast Quiche

We use quiches as our personal low-carbohydrate treat food. They are easy to make, great when they're still warm, and cold, straight from the refrigerator, they are great for eating when you're on the run. Best of all, they always make us say "ahhhh" when we bite into them. This is one of our favorites.

1 teaspoon olive oil	ground black pepper to taste
¼ cup heavy cream	
¼ pound Cheddar cheese, grated	2 eggs, lightly beaten
2 cups sliced mushrooms	1 cup chopped leftover cooked steak or chicken (optional)
1 cup diced cauliflower	
dash dried basil	½ package frozen spinach, thawed, liquid squeezed out
paprika to taste	

Preheat oven to 325°F.

Oil the bottom and sides of a 9-inch glass or ceramic pie pan or a glass or ceramic loaf pan.

In a medium saucepan, heat cream until hot, but do not let it boil. Remove from heat and quickly stir in grated cheese.

When cheese is melted, add mushrooms, cauliflower, basil, paprika, and pepper.

Cool for 5 minutes. Add one egg at a time, meat or chicken, and the spinach. Mix well after each addition.

Pour mixture into oiled pan and bake until custard is set, 45 to 50 minutes.

Herby Cream Cheese–Filled Mushrooms

We love to have these tasty little fellows for breakfast—or with lunch or dinner, or both, as well!

1 tablespoon olive oil	$\frac{1}{2}$ teaspoon fresh lemon juice
2 ounces cream cheese	
$\frac{1}{2}$ tablespoon heavy cream	$\frac{1}{4}$ teaspoon salt
	ground black pepper to taste
$\frac{1}{2}$ teaspoon minced fresh chives	
	8 large mushroom caps
$\frac{1}{2}$ teaspoon dried basil	paprika to taste

Preheat oven to 350°F.

Put olive oil in shallow baking pan and set aside.

In a small bowl, use a fork to combine cream cheese, cream, chives, basil, lemon juice, salt, and black pepper. Mix until smooth.

Spoon a generous amount of the mixture into each inverted mushroom cap and sprinkle lightly with paprika.

Place mushroom caps into the oiled pan and bake for 10 to 15 minutes.

Beefy Cream Cheese Roll-Up

SERVES 4

The one and only grocery store on Block Island, Rhode Island, was closed due to inclement weather, and these were all of the foods we had left in the house. We put these ingredients all together and came out with a recipe that was so good and so easy that we've been enjoying it ever since.

$^1/_2$ pound leftover cooked steak, rib roast, or other lean beef, cut into strips

$^1/_8$ teaspoon salt

$^1/_4$ teaspoon dry mustard, or to taste

4 ounces cream cheese

$^1/_4$ cup mayonnaise

1 tablespoon fresh lemon juice

$^1/_2$ tablespoon chopped pitted green olives

$^1/_2$ tablespoon chopped pitted black olives

$^1/_4$ teaspoon dried sweet basil ground black pepper to taste

8 large lettuce leaves, washed and patted dry chopped fresh chives

In a medium mixing bowl blend beef and salt. Add dry mustard as desired. Add cream cheese and mix until smooth.

Add mayonnaise, lemon juice, olives, basil, and black pepper. Divide the mixture into 8 equal portions.

On a lettuce leaf, lay down a portion of the beef mixture forming a strip lengthwise down the center.

Sprinkle the strip with some chopped chives and roll up the lettuce leaf.

Repeat this process for the remaining lettuce leaves.

Breakfast Pockets

Leftovers are a standard in our house. We cook extra portions to ensure that we have enough to enjoy later. We love to add cheese, or often substitute meat for the chicken, in this well-used recipe.

2 leftover baked chicken breasts	1 tablespoon chopped scallions
3 tablespoons white vinegar	4 tablespoons chopped spinach
½ cup olive oil	1 medium green bell pepper, finely diced
1 teaspoon Dijon mustard	
1 tablespoon chopped parsley	8 large spinach leaves, washed and patted dry

Chop the chicken into small chunks.

In a mixer, blend vinegar, olive oil, mustard, parsley, scallions, chopped spinach, and green pepper. Blend until smooth to make green salsa.

On the center of each spinach leaf, lay down a large spoonful of the chicken chunks.

Top the chicken with a large tablespoon of salsa.

Fold top and bottom, and both sides of the spinach leaf to form a pocket.

Hungarian Cheese Spread on Poached Salmon

SERVES 4

When we make poached salmon, we always make extra so that we can enjoy this dish the next morning. It's our variation on a special dish we tasted at a wedding brunch. We promised ourselves we would try it at home without the loud music.

4 romaine lettuce leaves, rinsed and patted dry

4 4-ounce pieces poached salmon (page 55)

4 ounces cream cheese

2 tablespoons olive oil

3 tablespoons sour cream

2 ounces feta cheese, crumbled

1 teaspoon prepared mustard

2 teaspoons dried basil

1 teaspoon hot paprika

1/4 teaspoon salt

1/2 teaspoon capers

Set out four plates and lay a lettuce leaf on each. Place a piece of salmon on each leaf.

In a medium bowl, mix together cream cheese and olive oil. Add sour cream, feta cheese, mustard, basil, paprika, and salt. Mix with a fork until smooth.

Spoon a quarter of the mixture over the top of each piece of salmon. Sprinkle with capers.

Poached Salmon

Everyone seems to think that poached salmon should take time and effort. We think it couldn't be easier and we bet you'll think so, too. When we have guests, Rachael uses cake decorating disks to make cream cheese flowers all around the fish.

2 tablespoons olive oil	¹⁄₄ cup white vinegar
4 tablespoons chopped garlic	salt to taste
¹⁄₄ cup chopped green bell pepper	white peppercorns to taste
¹⁄₄ cup chopped celery	1 large salmon fillet, about 1¹⁄₂ to 2 pounds
1 quart water	cheesecloth, if available

Combine olive oil, garlic, green pepper, and celery in large skillet. Sauté the mixture for 5 to 8 minutes. Add water, vinegar, salt, and peppercorns, and simmer for 5 minutes.

Bring liquid to boil as you wrap the salmon fillet in coarse cheesecloth (if available).

Submerge the salmon in boiling liquid. Immediately lower heat and allow fish to simmer for 25 to 30 minutes.

Remove salmon steak and carefully unwrap. (If you are not using cheesecloth, use two large spatulas to remove the fish.)

DIPS, DRESSINGS,
and
SAUCES

Dips and dressings and sauces, oh my! We love them and find that, too often, these lovely additions get lost in the low-carb, no-time-to-cook shuffle.

We think that dips, sauces, and dressings add taste, sparkle, and pizzazz. They're like the jewelry and makeup that finish off an outfit. No matter how hectic things get, we hope you will try to make time to take care of yourself and to light up your low-carb meals with some of the special tastes and flavors these welcome additions can provide.

Lemon-Lime Drizzle

*We invented this at a restaurant table when all the salad
dressings they had were unacceptable for a low-carb meal.
Our waitress liked it so much that she took the recipe home.
(We added the capers later).*

4 ounces extra virgin olive oil	⅛ teaspoon salt
	black pepper to taste
1 tablespoon fresh lemon juice, strained for seeds	1 tablespoon chopped fresh parsley
1 tablespoon fresh lime juice, strained for seeds	2 tablespoons capers

Combine all of the ingredients in a glass jar and shake
well.

Let the mixture stand for 15 minutes before using.

When ready, drizzle over steamed vegetables, such as
asparagus or cauliflower or use as a marinade for meat,
chicken, fish, or tofu.

Creamy Fresh Herb Dip

One of the best things about this dip is the fresh, clean flavor that makes it a great complement for almost any protein or vegetable dish.

2 cups sour cream

½ cup basil leaves, minced

¼ cup minced fresh chives

¼ cup minced green bell pepper

¼ cup minced fresh mint

1 teaspoon minced fresh cilantro

3 cloves garlic, minced

1 tablespoon teriyaki sauce*

salt to taste

black pepper to taste

Tabasco sauce to taste

Combine all the ingredients in a large bowl and blend well. Chill.

To serve, put into a serving dish and set on a large platter or flat basket or tray and surround with fresh, crisp raw cucumber, celery, green beans, and mushrooms.

*Most recent Carbohydrate Addict's books may contain alternative guidelines for this ingredient. Consult your book's food lists for guidance. Use acceptable alternative as appropriate.

Nondairy Cream Sauce

*Our wonderful friend and our support group administrator,
Barbara, is lactose intolerant. We developed this recipe so she
could enjoy the pleasure of a good creamy sauce.*

2 cups chopped cauliflower	$\frac{1}{2}$ tablespoon chopped fresh tarragon
1 clove garlic, quartered	2 tablespoons lime juice
2 tablespoons chopped fresh chives	2 tablespoons olive oil
1 tablespoon chopped fresh cilantro	$\frac{1}{4}$ cup puréed tofu (or light cream)
	salt to taste

In food processor fitted with chopping blade or appropriate blender, purée cauliflower with garlic, herbs, and lime
juice.

Place olive oil in a saucepan over low heat. Stir in
cauliflower purée and cook over low heat, stirring occasionally, until heated through. Add cream or tofu and
continue to heat, but do not allow to boil.

Salt to taste and serve.

No-Cook Cheddar Cheese Sauce

Whenever we crave something new and exciting to eat, we pull out this recipe. It's a interesting twist on plain old cheese sauce.

¼ cup crumbled Cheddar
   cheese
1 tablespoon white vinegar

¼ cup mayonnaise
½ cup heavy cream
⅛ teaspoon black pepper

In a blender, combine Cheddar cheese, vinegar, and mayonnaise.

With blender running, slowly add cream.

Season with pepper.

Cucumber Cloud Supreme

Our friend Lynn is a weaver. The clothes and wall hangings that she creates are soft and airy. She walks through life with sweetness and grace in the face of difficulty and challenge. It's no wonder that when we spent an extended weekend at her home, we discovered that the food she serves her family is also delicate and light.

3 medium cucumbers, peeled and seeded	1 tablespoon chopped fresh dill weed
1 teaspoon salt	1 tablespoon chopped fresh parsley
1 cup heavy cream	1 tablespoon chopped fresh chives
½ cup sour cream	

Grate cucumber and sprinkle with salt to help draw out the water.

Allow to drain in a colander or on paper towels for half an hour.

Beat cream until it begins to stiffen.

Fold in sour cream and herbs.

Press remaining moisture out of cucumber and fold into cream mixture.

Chill before serving.

Zippy Lemon Dressing

Our friend Alan is zippy and quick. He is the zesty balance to his wife's gentle being. It's no wonder that his favorite dressing is zippy and quick, too.

¹/₄ cup fresh lemon juice

1 tablespoon grated lemon zest

2 tablespoons chopped fresh dill weed

¹/₄ teaspoon salt

³/₄ cup olive oil

¹/₂ teaspoon dill seed

Beat all ingredients together until well blended. Chill and serve.

Spicy Egg Dressing/Dip

This recipe makes us think of some of our favorite camping trips. We always pack these ingredients because we know we can always throw this wonderful dish together without needing blenders or mixers or any kitchen appliances. Have whisk will travel!

2 egg yolks*
3 cloves garlic, mashed
   dash salt
³/₄ cup olive oil
¹/₂ teaspoon white vinegar

¹/₂ teaspoon fresh lemon juice

Tabasco or other hot sauce, to taste

Beat egg yolks until very thick and lemon colored.

Add mashed garlic and salt and beat again, adding olive oil drop by drop.

As the mixture thickens, add vinegar and lemon juice. Then continue adding olive oil slowly, beating until a thick emulsion is formed.

Add hot sauce to taste.

This mixture may be used as an alternative to mayonnaise or as a sauce or dip for seafood or vegetables.

*Use certified, salmonella-free eggs only.

Quick and Easy Hollandaise

Whenever we enjoy this sauce, one of us always smiles and remarks with impish delight, "Yes, isn't it tough to be on a diet!"

3 egg yolks	1 cup (¹/₂ pound) sweet butter
¹/₂ teaspoon salt	
dash cayenne pepper	1 tablespoon lemon juice
1 tablespoon heavy cream	

Place egg yolks, salt, cayenne, and cream in blender.

Blend for a few seconds at high speed until you have a smooth frothy mixture. Put aside.

Melt butter in small pan over low heat until bubbling but not brown.

With blender at high speed, start adding the hot butter in a thin, steady stream. As butter is added, the sauce will thicken.

When half the butter has been added, add lemon juice. Continue blending until all butter is used.

Sour Cream Dill Sauce

When we're under deadline and we don't want to give up the pleasures of a good and tasty sauce, we count on this recipe to meet all of our needs.

1/2 cup sour cream

1/2 cup mayonnaise

1/2 tablespoon finely minced garlic

1 tablespoon lime juice

2 tablespoons chopped fresh dill weed

Combine all ingredients and mix well. Chill.

Creamy Clam & Crab Dip

When Rachael was a teenager, her first baby-sitting job had this in the 'fridge. She's never forgotten it, though now we enjoy it with low-carb veggies.

8	ounces cream cheese, softened	1	6½-ounce can crabmeat, drained and minced
4	tablespoons olive oil	1	6½-ounce can clams, drained and minced
¼	cup mayonnaise		

In a saucepan over low to medium heat, combine all ingredients, stirring occasionally for about 30 minutes until warmed thoroughly.

Serve with sliced green peppers, cauliflower florets, mushrooms, and whole green beans.

Tangy Mustard Vinaigrette

We whip this up in a few minutes and throw it into a small jar or plastic container when we need to take a dressing on the road.

¼ cup white vinegar	2 teaspoons Dijon mustard
salt to taste	¾ cup olive oil
black pepper to taste	

In a small bowl, combine vinegar, salt, pepper, and mustard.

Blend in olive oil and let stand for 5 minutes; adjust seasoning as desired.

Pour into closed jar for storage. Shake before using.

Savory Sauce with Spices

Put four scientists in a kitchen and you get five opinions. On a recent vacation, when all the dust had settled, this creamy flavorful sauce was born. We love to spoon this mixture on warm or cold vegetables, meats, poultry, or seafood.

2 cups sour cream	1/2 teaspoon ground cinnamon
2 teaspoons ground cumin	1/4 teaspoon freshly ground black pepper
1 1/2 teaspoons ground coriander	1/4 teaspoon ground cloves
1 1/2 teaspoons ground cardamom	1/4 teaspoon ground mace
1/2 teaspoon ground ginger	1/4 teaspoon ground nutmeg

Combine all the ingredients in a medium bowl and mix well.

Transfer to an airtight container and refrigerate for 24 hours to let flavors blend.

Garlic-Lime Vinaigrette

When people say they want more variety in their low-carb meals, we ask them which sauces are they using. Most have never taken the time or energy to add sauces to their proteins or vegetables. We find that it makes all the difference in the world!

1 small clove garlic, finely minced	¼ cup extra virgin olive oil
¼ teaspoon coarse salt	¼ cup olive oil
½ teaspoon dry mustard	salt to taste
2 tablespoons fresh lime juice	black pepper to taste

In a bowl, whisk together the garlic, coarse salt, mustard, and lime juice.

Slowly pour in both olive oils, mixing constantly until thickened.

Season with salt and pepper.

Cover and refrigerate 1 or 2 days.

Bring to room temperature before using.

Roasted Green Pepper Sauce

SERVES 8

One of Richard's favorite Reward Meal condiments is a jelly made from green peppers. For low-carb meals, he enjoys this sauce that adds the same full flavor.

4	large green bell peppers	$1/2$	teaspoon salt
1	tablespoon olive oil	$1/2$	teaspoon dried thyme
$1^{1}/2$	tablespoons dry white wine	$1/4$	teaspoon crushed red pepper
$1/2$	cup minced chives	$1/4$	teaspoon black pepper
1	clove garlic, minced		

Preheat broiler.

Cut bell peppers in half lengthwise, discarding the seeds and membranes.

Cover a baking sheet with aluminum foil and grease with the olive oil.

Place pepper halves skin side up, then flatten with your hand.

Broil 15 minutes or until blackened.

Place the peppers in a heavy-duty zip-top plastic bag, seal, and let stand 15 minutes. Remove peppers, peel, and place in a food processor. Process until smooth. Set aside.

In a medium saucepan, combine wine, chives, and garlic and boil for 10 minutes.

Add wine mixture, salt, thyme, crushed red pepper, and black pepper to puréed bell pepper in processor, and process until smooth.

When ready to serve, heat and pour over your favorite cooked meat.

Horseradish Sauce

After we first made, and tasted, this recipe, we found a dozen different dishes to put it on.

½ cup mayonnaise

½ cup sour cream

2 tablespoons prepared white horseradish

1 teaspoon lemon juice

Place mayonnaise, sour cream, and horseradish in a bowl and stir well to mix.

Add lemon juice and blend in thoroughly.

Amazing Onion Dip

Our good friend Squigs loves premade packaged onion dip.
Here's a no-glutamate variation that keeps the flavors but loses
the carbohydrates.

2 tablespoons chopped onions	2 tablespoons olive oil
	1 cup sour cream

In a small frying pan, fry onion in olive oil until deep
brown.

Remove from heat and let cool.

When cooled, add sour cream.

Stir very well to ensure complete mixture of onions,
oil, and sour cream.

DIPS, DRESSINGS, AND SAUCES ❖ 73

Feta Vinaigrette

Our friend Donna is Armenian American. Her wonderful disposition shines through in all that she does, including this simple but flavorful salad dressing.

3 tablespoons olive oil	⅛ teaspoon Dijon mustard
1 tablespoon white vinegar	1 cup feta cheese, crumbled
1 large clove garlic, crushed	

Place all ingredients in small jar, close lid tightly and shake vigorously.

Let stand at least 24 hours to give garlic a chance to permeate the mixture.

Caesar Salad Dressing

We could eat Caesar salads day after day, but we save them for special occasions so that they remain new and exciting. Instead, we use this recipe to dress up simple broiled or baked meat, chicken, or fish dishes. Or we add it to tofu for a new and satisfying Caesarlike flavor.

1 egg*	½ teaspoon crushed red pepper
¾ cup olive oil	
¾ cup grated Parmesan cheese	4 teaspoons teriyaki sauce†
¼ cup lemon juice	½ teaspoon minced garlic
1 teaspoon salt	

Coddle the egg (boil shell-less in water for 1 minute), then put it in a blender and beat until fluffy.

Add olive oil in slow stream. Reduce speed and add remaining ingredients in order.

Store in refrigerator in glass jar or other appropriate covered container.

*Use certified, salmonella-free eggs only.
† Most recent Carbohydrate Addict's books may contain alternative guidelines for this ingredient. Consult your book's food lists for guidance. Use acceptable alternative as appropriate.

DIPS, DRESSINGS, AND SAUCES ❖ 75

Lemony Garlic Dressing

Rachael tells the story of her grandmother being away from her grandfather for the first weekend in forty years. Though she left him with every meal prepared and ready in the refrigerator, he took the opportunity to strike out on his own. Rachael and her brother pretended they loved his culinary creation so as not to hurt Grandpop's feelings. Later, as an adult, Rachael discovered the simple recipe that her grandfather had given to her so many years before. It was that much more precious because he did not have the ability to read or write and counted on her to save it for posterity. Surprisingly, we both discovered that as adults, we truly enjoyed the grown-up taste of this simple, old-world recipe.

1 clove garlic, minced	1 tablespoon lemon juice
1/2 teaspoon paprika	1/2 cup olive oil
1/2 teaspoon teriyaki sauce*	black pepper to taste
1/4 teaspoon ground cumin	

In a bowl, whisk together the minced garlic, paprika, teriyaki sauce, cumin, and lemon juice.

Gradually add olive oil, whisking constantly.

Blend in black pepper.

*Most recent Carbohydrate Addict's books may contain alternative guidelines for this ingredient. Consult your book's food lists for guidance. Use acceptable alternative as appropriate.

Cheese and Caraway Dip

We first tasted this dip while on a bus traveling through the outback in Australia. Two young Scandinavian women brought it along as traveler's dip for celery and green peppers. We were quite impressed to find that they naturally ate in such a healthy way although they knew nothing of carbohydrate addiction.

8 ounces cream cheese, softened	2 teaspoons paprika
¹/₂ cup olive oil	1 teaspoon caraway seed
3 tablespoons sour cream	¹/₂ teaspoon salt
3 cloves garlic, minced	4 ounces feta cheese
1 tablespoon prepared mustard	2 anchovy fillets
	1 teaspoon capers, drained

In a large mixing bowl, combine all ingredients except anchovy fillets and capers.

Blend well and chill for 2 hours.

Transfer mixture to a serving plate, shape into a smooth mound, and garnish with anchovy fillets and capers.

More sour cream can be added to adjust dipping consistency.

Green Spinach Sauce

*If Popeye were entertaining, this is surely what he'd serve
with raw green beans, green peppers, mushrooms, and sliced
cucumbers.*

1 cup sour cream	¼ cup chopped parsley
1 cup fresh spinach, stems removed	salt to taste
1 large clove garlic, minced	black pepper to taste

Put sour cream into blender with spinach, minced garlic,
and parsley and then purée.

Pour into a bowl and season to taste.

BEEF and VEAL

For us, there is nothing like having a special meat meal. We know our feelings are not shared by everyone, and we love our tofu-based meals as well, but for us a special meat meal can really satisfy.

We always choose lean cuts and vary our diets with meals that include poultry and seafood and tofu as well but, when a beef or veal dish is on the menu, we know we're in for a special treat.

Veal Marsala Burgers

We love gourmet burgers made from ground meat with savory ingredients that transform them into fancy treats.

½ teaspoon minced garlic	½ pound ground veal
3 fresh parsley sprigs, stems removed	2 tablespoons olive oil
1 egg	2 tablespoons dry Marsala wine
½ teaspoon dried sage	2 tablespoons sour cream
½ teaspoon dried tarragon	ground black pepper to taste
½ tablespoon dried basil	

In a blender, combine garlic, parsley, egg, sage, tarragon, and basil. Blend quickly to combine without making the texture too fine.

Place veal in a small bowl and add herb mixture slowly, incorporating mixture into meat.

Place meat mixture on a piece of wax paper.

Form veal into 4 small, flat cakes. Set aside.

Place olive oil in a sauté pan or skillet over high heat.

Add veal patties, lower heat, and cook until dark golden brown, about 4 minutes on each side.

Pour Marsala into pan and stir.

Cook for one more minute, remove from heat, and allow to cool.

Add sour cream to sauce. Stir well.

Season to taste with pepper.

Peppery Quick Filet Mignon

Rachael's father made two dishes: scrambled eggs and peppery steak. Here's our updated version of her childhood favorite.

- 2 tablespoons sesame oil
- ½ teaspoon hot pepper flakes
- 3 tablespoons green peppercorns
- 3 tablespoons black peppercorns
- 4 4-ounce beef tenderloin steaks, 1 inch thick, trimmed

Combine sesame oil and hot pepper flakes and store overnight in airtight container.

When ready to prepare meal, firmly press peppercorns into steaks.

Brush pepper oil on steaks and place steaks in a medium nonstick skillet.

Cook 1 minute on each side over high heat.

Reduce heat to medium and cook 7 minutes per side, or until desired degree of doneness is reached.

Creamy Veal Chops

SERVES 4

Since veal chops can be more expensive than other cuts of beef, when we have it, we like to make it into a memorable and elegant dish.

3	tablespoons olive oil	1	cup heavy cream
4	veal chops		salt to taste
2	tablespoons dry white wine		black pepper to taste

Put olive oil into a heavy skillet over high heat.

Add veal chops and brown, about 3 minutes on each side.

Add white wine to the pan. Cook for 1 minute.

Add cream and stir in all the brown bits and juices.

Add salt and pepper, cover the skillet, lower the heat, and continue cooking for 15 to 20 minutes, or until chops are tender.

Remove the chops to a hot serving dish and serve immediately.

Beef Provençal Stuffed with Mushrooms

SERVES 4

Toronto is known for its metropolitan restaurants. Right across from our hotel, we found a little restaurant with only five or six tables. The owner cooked, served, and cleaned up. This version of his "house beef" proves that if you want to do something right, it pays to do it yourself.

4 4-ounce beef filet steaks, pounded thin for rolling

2 tablespoons sesame oil

1 clove garlic, minced

½ cup minced scallions

6 ounces mushroom caps, chopped

salt to taste

black pepper to taste

2 tablespoons chopped fresh parsley

1 4-ounce chunk mozzarella cheese, quartered lengthwise

2 tablespoons olive oil

1 teaspoon teriyaki sauce*

Preheat oven to 400°F.

In a large skillet over medium heat, brown steaks in sesame oil on both sides. Remove steaks and put aside.

In same skillet, combine garlic and scallions and cook, stirring, until scallions are soft, 2 to 3 minutes.

Add the mushrooms and cook, stirring, until soft, about 4 minutes.

Season to taste with salt and pepper, add the parsley, and remove from heat.

Place ¼ of mushroom mixture and 1 piece of mozzarella cheese on each filet.

Roll up filets and secure with wooden toothpicks.

Place filets, seam side down, on cookie sheet lightly oiled with olive oil.

Sprinkle with teriyaki sauce and bake for 20 minutes, until cooked through.

Remove toothpicks and serve immediately.

*Most recent Carbohydrate Addict's books may contain alternative guidelines for this ingredient. Consult your book's food lists for guidance. Use acceptable alternative as appropriate.

Basic Prime Rib

Rachael never knew the difference between prime rib and roast beef until she had this recipe. No wonder they call it "prime."

1 4-pound prime rib roast	black pepper to taste
water	½ teaspoon dried rosemary
salt to taste	

Preheat oven to 500°F.

Place the rib roast in roasting pan on roasting rack. Add water to pan, but do not let the water touch the meat.

Season meat with salt, pepper, and rosemary, and sear in oven for 15 minutes.

Lower heat to 350°F and cook until internal temperature reaches correct level as indicated on meat thermometer (approximately 135°F for rare; 155°F for medium—30 to 45 minutes per pound).

Remove roast from oven, cover with a sheet of foil, and let rest for about 10 minutes.

When ready to serve, set the roast, rib side down, on a cutting board and cut into thick or thin slices.

For thin slices, cut meat off the ribs. For thick ones, cut between the ribs as necessary.

Remove and save water, now flavored with drippings, for gravy.

To thicken gravy, pour flavored drippings into a saucepan and cook down.

Herby Beef Tenderloin

We have found that vinegar and oil bring out the subtle flavors of herbs and spices not only in salad dressings but in cooked dishes as well. This is a trusted standby for us.

1½ pounds beef tenderloin, center cut, trimmed

8 large spinach leaves, washed, and patted dry

1½ tablespoons white vinegar

8 tablespoons olive oil

½ tablespoon dried rosemary

½ tablespoon dried sage

salt to taste

ground black pepper to taste

Cut the tenderloin into 12 medallions, each about ¾ inch thick.

Between two pieces of waxed paper, gently pound the meat until it is ¼ inch thick.

Arrange spinach leaves on a large serving platter and drizzle with the vinegar and 5 tablespoons of the oil.

Brush two large skillets with 1 tablespoon of oil each. Sear the tenderloin medallions until cooked, about 3 minutes on each side.

Put medallion in a single layer over the spinach and sprinkle with crumbled rosemary, sage, salt, and pepper, and the remaining tablespoon olive oil.

Grilled Steaks and Garlic

Hot steak, cold steak, it's good at any temperature. We make up several steaks at the same time, cut them up, bag them, refrigerate or freeze them, and enjoy them time after time.

½ cup olive oil	4 cloves garlic, chopped
½ cup chopped cilantro	½ cup lime juice
1 teaspoon black pepper, or to taste	6 4-ounce sirloin steaks

In a large bowl, combine olive oil, cilantro, black pepper, garlic, and lime juice.

Add steaks and turn to coat the meat.

Refrigerate at least 4 hours. Can be refrigerated overnight.

Prepare barbecue (medium heat) or electric grill.

Carefully pour marinade over uncooked meat prior to placing on grill.

Grill steaks until done to your desire.

Steak in a Blanket

We often depend on the flavor and pleasure of this dish to make our breakfast or lunch a satisfying experience.

2	teaspoons white vinegar	$^2/_3$	teaspoon olive oil
1	cup chopped cauliflower	1	medium green bell pepper, chopped
2	teaspoons teriyaki sauce*		salt to taste
1	large clove garlic, minced		black pepper to taste
$^1/_2$	small jalapeño chile pepper, seeded and minced	12	leaves romaine lettuce, rinsed and drained
1	pound flank steak, pounded thin		

Preheat broiler.

In a medium bowl, mix vinegar, cauliflower, teriyaki sauce, garlic, and jalapeño.

Add flank steak and turn to coat the meat. Let stand in refrigerator for 15 minutes to marinate.

Remove flank steak from the marinade, transfer to a broiling pan lined with aluminum foil and broil 3 minutes on each side, until thoroughly done.

Transfer flank steak to a carving board and let stand for 5 minutes.

Heat olive oil in a nonstick skillet. Add green pepper and sauté until softened, about 6 minutes. Season with salt and pepper to taste.

Cutting at an angle, slice flank steak across the grain into $^1/_4$-inch-thick slices.

Arrange a slice of the flank steak on each lettuce leaf and top with a portion of the cauliflower mixture. Roll each lettuce leaf around meat and filling and serve immediately.

---

*Most recent Carbohydrate Addict's books may contain alternative guidelines for this ingredient. Consult your book's food lists for guidance. Use acceptable alternative as appropriate.

Crock-Pot Roast

As winter approaches and the days grow shorter, we pull out our Crock-Pot. On days when work requires a Reward Meal lunch, we place a new protein and vegetable combination into the Crock-Pot to cook and, when we return in the evening, a warm and welcoming low-carbohydrate dinner like this is waiting to greet us.

1 pound beef pot roast	salt to taste
2 cloves garlic, cut into thin slivers	black pepper to taste
	4 medium parsley sprigs

Wash pot roast and lay in Crock-Pot, fat side down.

Lay garlic slivers over the top of the roast and sprinkle lightly with salt and pepper.

Set dial on low and cook, covered, about 4 or 5 hours or until thoroughly done.

Check to see if the meat pulls apart easily.

Serve the meat with some of the cooking juices and sprigs of parsley on top.

Mel Burgers

We love this variation and depend on it almost as much as much as we do on our good friend, Mel.

1 small onion, diced	4 ounces spicy all-beef sausage meat, removed from casings
2 tablespoons olive oil	
2 pounds ground beef	2 large eggs

In frying pan, sauté diced onion in olive oil until onion turns dark brown.

Remove from heat and cool.

In a large bowl, combine the onion and the oil they cooked in with the rest of the ingredients.

Form into patties.

Return patties to frying pan or cook on grill or under broiler until done.

Perfect with Molly's Mushrooms (page 229), and a sugarless dill pickle, too!

Tom's Surprise Burgers

When a burger's cheese remains inside, it retains its full flavor and texture. The exquisite taste of this favorite of ours may surprise you.

1 pound ground beef	½ teaspoon dried tarragon
4 ounces sausage meat, removed from casings	2 large eggs
	1 teaspoon teriyaki sauce*
½ teaspoon powdered garlic	6 slices mozzarella cheese
½ teaspoon dried basil	

Combine all ingredients except cheese.

Form into 12 very thin patties.

Place one slice of mozzarella cheese between two patties. Seal so that meat covers all cheese.

Cook on electric or outdoor grill, pan fry in olive oil, or cook under broiler until done.

*Most recent Carbohydrate Addict's books may contain alternative guidelines for this ingredient. Consult your book's food lists for guidance. Use acceptable alternative as appropriate.

Celery Steak Stir-Fry

SERVES 6

Most people overcook celery and don't realize how good it can be. Be sure to stir-fry the celery quickly. When you sauté the celery lightly, its subtle flavor and texture can add a whole new dimension to your meal. This is delicious with raw mushrooms and low-carb dip.

2 cloves garlic, chopped	1½ pounds round steak, cut into bite-size chunks
3 tablespoons olive oil	
2 tablespoons teriyaki sauce*	salt to taste
6 celery stalks, cleaned, and cut into bite-size chunks	pepper to taste

In a large skillet over medium heat, sauté garlic in olive oil.

Stir in teriyaki sauce and, when warmed, add celery. Sauté, stirring constantly for about 5 minutes. Remove celery and set aside.

Add steak chunks and brown on all sides. Cook until steak is fully done, stirring often.

Add celery, stir for a moment or two to heat.

Season with salt and pepper and serve.

*Most recent Carbohydrate Addict's books may contain alternative guidelines for this ingredient. Consult your book's food lists for guidance. Use acceptable alternative as appropriate.

Left Bank Burgers

We never thought we would find the perfect American burger in Paris, but we did—in a sidewalk cafe that sold hot dogs, burgers, and "American Fries"!

1	pound ground beef	1	teaspoon salt
½	cup heavy cream	1	tablespoon diced garlic
1	tablespoon dry sherry	½	teaspoon ground sage
2	eggs	1	tablespoon dried parsley

Preheat broiler.
  Combine all ingredients.
  Form into four thick patties.
  Broil for 5 to 8 minutes per side.

Basic Steak and Peppers

SERVES 4

*When she was a little girl, Rachael had a dog, Blaze, who loved
this dish. He once ate up the whole batch of steaks and peppers
that had been left to cool. His breath smelled like green peppers
for days afterward.*

1/4 cup olive oil

1 pound minute steaks

2 whole green bell peppers,
cored and cut into 1/2-inch
slices

1/2 cup water

1 tablespoon chopped fresh
basil

1 teaspoon thyme,
crumbled

1 tablespoon chopped
fresh parsley

1 bay leaf

salt to taste

pepper to taste

Preheat oven to 350°F.

Heat olive oil in skillet over medium heat.

Quickly brown steaks in olive oil, then remove steaks
to a shallow covered baking dish.

In hot pan, sauté peppers in oil until limp. Transfer
peppers to baking dish.

Return pan to medium heat.

Add water, herbs, and bay leaf to pan, scrape browned
bits into mixture as it heats. Pour mixture over steak and
peppers.

Cover baking dish, place in oven, and bake for 30 to 35
minutes, basting once or twice during cooking.

Remove bay leaf.

Add salt and pepper and serve warm.

Peking Stir-Fried Beef

We invented this dish on the spot when we realized we were obligated to join a group of colleagues intent on eating at the local Chinese restaurant. We requested the help of the chef, whose sister, it turned out, was on one of our programs. Our friends thought that our food was a lot more appealing than the cornstarch-thickened dishes that our companions had for lunch.

3	tablespoons dry sherry	1	teaspoon olive oil
2	tablespoons dark sesame oil	³/₄	pound asparagus, cut into 1-inch pieces
1	tablespoon grated gingerroot	¹/₂	green bell pepper, cut into thin strips
1	tablespoon minced garlic	2	tablespoons teriyaki sauce*
1	pound sirloin steak, trimmed and cut into thin strips	¹/₂	pound whole fresh green beans, ends trimmed

In a large bowl combine sherry, sesame oil, gingerroot, and garlic. Add steak strips and let marinate 15 minutes.

Heat a wok over medium-high heat and add olive oil.

Stir-fry asparagus and bell pepper for 2 minutes, then remove to a platter.

Add steak and marinade to wok and stir-fry for 3 minutes.

Add teriyaki sauce and cook for 1 minute.

Return asparagus/pepper mixture to wok and cook for 1 minute, stirring constantly. Toss in green beans, cover wok, and cook for 1 minute. Serve immediately.

*Most recent Carbohydrate Addict's books may contain alternative guidelines for this ingredient. Consult your book's food lists for guidance. Use acceptable alternative as appropriate.

Crusty Beef Roast

We have found that when it comes to roasts, the cut is really important. Try a variety of cuts until you find one that's just right and make note of it. When we freeze the leftover meat, we include some of the juices in the plastic freezer bags.

2 cloves garlic, crushed	½ teaspoon dried tarragon, crushed
1 teaspoon salt	
1 teaspoon cracked black pepper	3 pound beef roast
	water
1 teaspoon dried thyme	¼ cup finely chopped scallion

Preheat oven to 350°F.

In a small bowl, combine garlic, salt, pepper, thyme, and tarragon to form a paste.

Rub the paste evenly over surface of the roast.

Place roast, fat side up, on rack in roasting pan. Fill bottom of pan with 1 or 2 inches of water; water should not touch meat. Lay scallions in water.

Insert meat thermometer into thickest part of roast, not touching fat or bone. Roast until thermometer registers 135°F for rare; 155°F for medium.

Cover roast with aluminum foil tent and allow to stand 15 to 20 minutes. Trim excess fat from roast before carving.

Serve roast with pan drippings.

Spicy Olive Burgers

If you like tangy hot foods, you'll enjoy the added zip that the jalapeño cheese provides in this recipe.

1½ pounds ground beef	2 tablespoons olive oil
3 ounces jalapeño cheese, crumbled	salt to taste
	black pepper to taste
3 tablespoons sliced olives, green or black	6 lettuce leaves

Divide ground beef into 12 equal portions and shape into very thin patties.

Place equal amounts of cheese and olives in center of 6 patties.

Top with remaining 6 patties, crimping the edges together to seal.

Heat olive oil in a large skillet over medium heat and cook patties for 5 to 6 minutes per side.

Season with salt and pepper.

Arrange 1 lettuce leaf on each plate and top each with 1 burger.

Serve immediately.

Far East Beef Teriyaki

The flavors blend after cooking when the leftovers are refrigerated overnight, so be sure to make extra to serve cold the next day.

1 pound sirloin steak, cut into 1-inch cubes

2 small green bell peppers, cut into 1-inch pieces

$^1\!/_2$ pound mushroom caps

teriyaki sauce to taste*

Place beef, green pepper, mushroom caps, and teriyaki sauce in a bowl. Turn meat and vegetables to coat well with sauce. Cover and refrigerate for at least an hour.

Thread the cubes of meat onto short bamboo skewers and grill very quickly over glowing coals on a barbecue or a hibachi. The meat should be placed about 4 inches away from the coals, and turned frequently.

The concept of a good teriyaki is to have the thin edges of the meat actually singed and beginning to get crisp while the center is still quite rare.

Thread mushroom caps and green peppers on skewers and place on grill when meat is about half done. Continue to cook until done throughout.

*Most recent Carbohydrate Addict's books may contain alternative guidelines for this ingredient. Consult your book's food lists for guidance. Use acceptable alternative as appropriate.

LAMB

New Zealand and lamb—the best of the best. Green hills roll past as we sit in the front of the bus, holding hands and watching the world go by. Each year we return to New Zealand for good food, good friends, and the time to enjoy both.

Frontier Pan-Broiled Lamb Chops

Rachael likes these chops almost burned. She adores the crusty crunch. Most people like them cooked to a bit more traditional doneness.

2 tablespoons olive oil

2 large lamb chops, 1 inch thick

¼ teaspoon garlic powder

salt to taste

black pepper to taste

Heat olive oil in a medium skillet over medium heat. When oil is hot, add chops.

Cook chops about 7 minutes on each side, turning chops only once. Season with garlic, salt, and pepper just before removing.

Stir pan juices, scraping pan. Pour juice over chops and serve hot.

Tarragon Lamb

The secret to keeping these chops crisp is spreading the chops apart as much as possible so that the heat sears them on all surfaces.

1	small 8-chop rack of lamb, about 1½ pounds	1	tablespoon dried thyme
1	large clove garlic, slivered	1	tablespoon coarsely ground black pepper
2	tablespoons olive oil	1	teaspoon coarse salt
2	tablespoons dried tarragon		

Preheat oven to 500°F.

Make deep slits all over the lamb and insert the garlic slivers.

Brush the chops lightly with olive oil.

In a medium bowl, combine tarragon, thyme, pepper, and salt and pat all over the lamb.

Place the lamb, fat side up, in a roasting pan. Insert meat thermometer from side; avoid touching the bone. Roast for 10 minutes.

Reduce the heat to 400°F and roast another 20 to 30 minutes depending on desired doneness as indicated by appearance of meat and meat thermometer.

Remove from the oven and let rest for 5 minutes before carving.

Serve immediately.

Creamy and Herby Leg of Lamb

SERVES 8

We adore the luscious creamy sauce that you make with this recipe. We think that you and your guests will like it, too.

1 6½-pound leg of lamb	1 cup dry white wine or water
4 cloves garlic, slivered	¼ cup heavy cream
2 tablespoons olive oil	½ cup sour cream
1 tablespoon dried oregano	½ teaspoon dried basil
1 tablespoon coarsely ground pepper	

Preheat oven to 400°F.

Place the leg of lamb in a large roasting pan and insert a meat thermometer; avoid touching the bone.

Cut deep slits over the surface of the lamb with the tip of a small sharp knife. Carefully insert the garlic slivers into the slits. Brush the surface of the meat with olive oil.

In a small bowl, combine the oregano and pepper.

Rub the mixture all over the lamb and pour the wine (or water) into the bottom of the pan.

Place the pan into the oven and reduce the heat to 350°F.

Roast, basting occasionally, about 1½ hours. The meat thermometer should read 175°F.

Let rest for 10 minutes before carving.

In a medium bowl, add cream to 1 cup of pan juice. Stir well. Add sour cream and basil. Stir well again.

The rest of the pan juices can be heated and served alongside the alternate creamy sauce.

Saucy Ground Lamb

Ground lamb and mint make a wonderfully fragrant combination. We discovered the inspiration for this dish while trekking through New Zealand, where the sheep outnumber the human inhabitants more than 10 to 1.

1 pound lamb, finely ground	7 tablespoons olive oil
4 medium cloves garlic, minced	salt to taste
	black pepper to taste
¾ cup fresh mint, minced	2 medium eggs
2 tablespoons minced fresh sage	1 tablespoon crushed green peppercorns
	¼ cup heavy cream

In a small bowl, combine the lamb, half of the garlic, the mint, sage, 4 tablespoons oil, salt, black pepper, and eggs. Mix well, cover, and refrigerate for at least 3 hours.

Divide mixture into 8 portions and form into patties.

Place 2 tablespoons olive oil in a large skillet over medium heat and add 4 patties. Cook for 3 minutes per side.

Repeat with the remaining 4 patties.

While the patties cook, place the remaining 1 tablespoon olive oil in a saucepan.

Add the remaining garlic and sauté until fragrant, about 30 seconds. Remove from heat and stir in peppercorns.

Add cream, stir very well, and cover to keep warm while lamb patties cook.

Place patties on plates, top with sauce, and serve.

Mediterranean Shish Kebab

With the radio thumping out the rhythm and a beat in our hearts, we threw together this hearty recipe. After the first bite, we ran to find a piece of paper to write down the ingredients and directions before we forgot them.

2 pounds leg of lamb, cubed for kebabs	$\frac{1}{8}$ teaspoon salt
$\frac{1}{2}$ cup olive oil	$\frac{1}{8}$ teaspoon ground black pepper
2 tablespoons fresh lemon juice	$\frac{1}{8}$ teaspoon dried oregano
3 large cloves garlic, peeled and crushed	$\frac{1}{8}$ teaspoon dried rosemary
1 teaspoon dry white wine	1 large green bell pepper, cut into 8 pieces
1 small bay leaf	12 medium mushroom caps

Place lamb in a large container with a cover.

In a medium bowl mix olive oil, lemon juice, garlic, wine, bay leaf, salt, pepper, oregano, and rosemary.

Pour marinade over lamb cubes and stir thoroughly. Cover and refrigerate, for at least 24 hours, stirring occasionally.

About 1 hour before serving, preheat broiler and drain lamb, reserving marinade.

(continued on next page)

Thread lamb, green pepper, and mushrooms on three separate skewers and place on a broiling tray. Baste vegetables with some of reserved marinade.

Broil about 4 inches from heat, turning frequently. Allow 6 to 8 minutes for the lamb, 3 to 4 minutes for the green peppers, and 2 to 3 minutes for the mushrooms.

Remove from broiler and allow to cool slightly, until ingredients and skewers can be handled. Leave broiler on.

Remove skewers from ingredients and rethread 4 to 8 skewers, alternating lamb, green pepper, and mushrooms.

Baste again with any remaining marinade.

Return skewers to broiler and, turning frequently, broil until meat is reheated and cooked medium-rare and vegetables are slightly blackened in spots.

Serve immediately.

Herbed Leg of Lamb

*Robin and Gavin took us into their hearts and their home—
a house blessed with beauty and love and with Jo-anne and
Matthew, their marvelous kids. We met in the Bake-Haus in
Cairns, Australia, where Robin works. They welcomed us with
great cooking and a generosity that we have rarely experienced.*

2 cloves garlic, slivered	1 teaspoon dried rosemary
1/3 cup olive oil	1/2 teaspoon dried thyme
1 teaspoon dried basil	3 pounds leg of lamb,
1 teaspoon salt	trimmed and cubed
1/2 teaspoon black pepper	

In a medium bowl combine garlic, olive oil, basil, salt, pepper, rosemary, and thyme.

Add lamb cubes to bowl and mix thoroughly to cover.

Cover and refrigerate for 30 minutes.

Preheat oven to 350°F.

Place lamb cubes on an aluminum foil–covered baking sheet and pour on the marinade.

Bake until cooked thoroughly but not overdone, about 1 hour.

Turn cubes to coat with pan juices once or twice during cooking.

Serve warm with the pan juices.

PORK

We used to think of pork as the "snack food" of meats—bacon, sausage, and ham for sandwiches. Now we have discovered that lean pork can be used in the best gourmet recipes (and those once-in-a-while old favorites still make us smile).

Paprika Pork Chops

SERVES 4

There are many kinds of paprikas available that add a wide variety of flavors to recipes. If you can find a good ethnic grocery, you can choose a paprika that seems to have the right taste for you. Don't be afraid to use it liberally. Most people think that paprika should be sprinkled on the surface of meats and poultry to enhance browning, but in many parts of Europe it is used as an essential seasoning.

4 large pork chops, ½ inch thick	1 tablespoon garlic powder
1 tablespoon teriyaki sauce*	1 tablespoon ground ginger
2 tablespoons olive oil	½ teaspoon paprika

Preheat oven to 375°F.

Trim fat from pork chops, and brush meat with teriyaki sauce.

Line a shallow baking dish with aluminum foil and coat the foil with olive oil. Place the pork chops in the dish.

In a small bowl, combine garlic, ginger, and paprika. Sprinkle ½ of this spice mixture on the chops.

Bake the chops, or cook on a grill, for 10 minutes.

Turn chops, coat with remaining spice mixture, and bake until cooked thoroughly but not overdone, about another 10 minutes.

Serve hot.

*Most recent Carbohydrate Addict's books may contain alternative guidelines for this ingredient. Consult your book's food lists for guidance. Use acceptable alternative as appropriate.

Simple Mustardy Pork Chops

These no muss–no fuss chops are made special by the flavor of browned garlic and the zing of the mustard glaze.

2	tablespoons olive oil	salt to taste	
1	teaspoon garlic, minced	pepper to taste	
4	pork chops, approximately 1 inch thick	¼ cup Dijon mustard	

Preheat oven to 350°F.

Heat 1 tablespoon olive oil in a skillet over medium heat.

Brown the garlic.

Add chops and continue to cook quickly over medium-high heat until they begin to brown, adding remaining 1 tablespoon oil to keep chops from sticking.

Season with salt and pepper to taste. Remove from heat and place chops on a cookie sheet.

Add mustard to the garlic and oil in skillet. Stir well as mixture cools.

Liberally spread half the mustard-garlic mixture onto one side of the chops.

Bake for 25 minutes.

Turn the chops and brush the other side with the remaining mustard-garlic mixture.

Return to oven and continue cooking for an additional 25 minutes or until thoroughly cooked.

Serve warm.

Tangy Pork Chops

SERVES 4

Mary Beth manages to care for her two little ones, her busy husband, and her career as a singer and stunt woman at Walt Disney World. It's a crazy life but she holds nothing back. We wish she knew how much she is appreciated. This wonderful recipe graces her table when she makes her annual pre-Christmas dinner for friends and family.

¼ cup chopped onion	1 clove garlic, crushed
2 tablespoons chopped fresh parsley	½ teaspoon dried thyme, crushed
2 tablespoons white vinegar	4 boneless center-cut pork rib chops, 1 inch thick
1 tablespoon olive oil	
2 teaspoons prepared mustard	

In a medium bowl, combine all ingredients except pork, blending well.

Place pork in plastic bag and add contents of the bowl. Turning to coat the meat well.

Close bag securely and marinate in refrigerator 6 to 8 hours or overnight. Turn occasionally to assure uniform marinating.

Preheat the broiler.

Remove pork chops from plastic bag and discard marinade.

Place pork chops on aluminum foil–covered baking sheet approximately 3 to 5 inches from heat. Broil chops 8 to 10 minutes per side.

Serve warm.

Sumptuous Pork Salad

Our best-bet salad made from leftovers.

2 cups cooked pork roast,
cut into bite-size pieces

1 cup diced celery

1 cup diced cauliflower

1 tablespoon Dijon mustard

3 tablespoons mayonnaise

Combine all ingredients and stir well. Serve on a bed of lettuce.

Shanghai Pork Roast

We use the cooked gravy from this wonderful recipe to quickly stir-fry some low-carb vegetables and make the meal complete.

2 tablespoons olive oil	½ teaspoon ground thyme
2 cloves garlic, minced	1 2-pound pork roast
½ teaspoon dried rosemary	1 cup water
	2 teaspoons teriyaki sauce*

Preheat oven to 350°F.

Mix oil, garlic, and herbs and rub all over pork roast.

Place roast in a shallow pan.

Combine water and teriyaki and pour over the roast.

Bake for 30 to 35 minutes per pound of meat, basting periodically, until meat thermometer registers 175°F.

Let the meat rest 10 minutes before carving.

*Most recent Carbohydrate Addict's books may contain alternative guidelines for this ingredient. Consult your book's food lists for guidance. Use acceptable alternative as appropriate.

New Age Stuffed Pork Chops

Richard likes to save this recipe for a low-carb dinner; it's filling and satisfying and perfect on a day you have a Reward Meal breakfast or lunch.

1 tablespoon olive oil	¼ teaspoon salt
1 cup fresh mushrooms, finely chopped	¼ teaspoon dried thyme
	¼ teaspoon pepper
¼ cup minced scallions	2 pounds pork chops, cut 2 inches thick and trimmed of excess fat
1 tablespoon dry red wine	

Heat olive oil in a heavy nonstick skillet over medium-high heat.

Add mushrooms and scallions and cook 4 to 5 minutes, stirring occasionally.

Add wine and cook an additional 5 minutes.

Add salt, thyme, and pepper.

Remove from heat and cool thoroughly.

Preheat broiler.

Cut a horizontal pocket into each chop, parallel to surface of meat, approximately 1 inch from each surface. Be careful not to cut all the way through to the opposite side.

Spoon cooled mushroom mixture into the pocket, spreading evenly. Use a wooden toothpick to secure the edge of each chop, in meat away from the side that will face the flame.

Place the chops on a broiler pan 5 inches from heat source.

Broil for 45 minutes, turning once during the broiling process.

Remove the chops and place on a warm serving platter.

Cover with aluminum foil and allow to stand 10 to 15 minutes.

Be certain to remove toothpicks before serving.

Roasted Pork with Rosemary and Garlic

The rosemary in this recipe brings a special aromatic flavor that makes the gravy taste uniquely satisfying.

2 tablespoons olive oil	2 tablespoons minced fresh rosemary
4 cloves garlic, peeled and halved	½ cup dry white wine, or water
1 3-pound pork roast	

Preheat oven to 350°F.

In a large ovenproof skillet over medium-high heat, heat olive oil and sauté garlic for 2 minutes.

Add pork roast to pan and brown lightly on all sides. Add rosemary to pan. Insert meat thermometer into center of the roast.

Cover skillet and bake until temperature exceeds 175°F, 65 to 70 minutes.

Remove roast to a platter and keep warm in the oven.

Add the wine (or water) to the skillet, and place the skillet over medium-high heat on the stove.

Scrape pan to loosen the browned bits in the skillet and blend with the liquid.

Cook rapidly for 2 to 3 minutes. Pour sauce over pork and serve.

POULTRY

Someday we'd love to write a cookbook called *One Hundred and One Ways to Cook a Chicken* (hopefully, not the same chicken)! We love recipes that call for all kinds of poultry because poultry takes on the flavor of whatever ingredients you add.

It's an old joke between us that, as we sit down to a meal of chicken, one of us says "Hmmm, tastes just like chicken," then we both smile. (Oh well, some couples are just like that!)

Chicken in a Garden

Sometimes something as small as a squirt of citrus flavor can add zest to a whole dish. Sometimes something as simple as little unexpected hugs and kind words can do the same for a relationship. We try to remind each other to include both in our cooking and in our lives.

½ cup olive oil

3 tablespoons lemon juice

2 teaspoons grated lemon zest

4 cloves garlic, peeled and sliced

8 fresh rosemary sprigs

salt to taste

black pepper to taste

1 medium roasting chicken, approximately 3 pounds, rinsed well and patted dry

2 cups cauliflower florets

2 cups broccoli florets*

In a large bowl, combine the olive oil, lemon juice and zest, garlic, rosemary, salt, and pepper.

Use this mixture to coat the chicken well. Cover and refrigerate overnight.

Preheat the oven to 400°F.

Remove the chicken from the marinade and place it in a large roasting pan.

Put the rosemary sprigs and garlic from the marinade into the cavity of the chicken. Pour the marinade over the chicken.

Roast the chicken for 55 minutes, basting occasionally.

Remove pan from the oven, arrange the cauliflower and broccoli around the chicken, and return the pan to the oven for an additional 5 minutes.

Remove the pan from the oven and let the chicken rest a few minutes before carving.

*Most recent Carbohydrate Addict's books may contain alternative guidelines for this ingredient. Consult your book's food lists for guidance. Use acceptable alternative as appropriate.

Spicy Chicken

SERVES 8

Low-carbohydrate meals shouldn't be bland or boring. We depend on spices and herbs and we try to mix unusual blends for new and surprising tastes.

8 boneless, skinless chicken breast halves

1 cup chopped chives

¼ cup fresh thyme leaves

2 tablespoons olive oil

1 tablespoon freshly ground pepper

1 tablespoon freshly ground coriander seeds

3 tablespoons grated peeled gingerroot

2 tablespoons fresh lime juice

2 teaspoons salt

2 teaspoons freshly ground allspice

1 teaspoon freshly ground nutmeg

1 teaspoon ground cinnamon

2 cloves garlic, peeled and halved

3 bay leaves

Place chicken in a large, shallow nonstick baking pan and set aside.

Put all the remaining ingredients into the container of a blender or food processor and process until a paste forms. If it becomes too thick, add a drop or two of olive oil until a "rubbing" consistency is obtained.

Rub this paste over both sides of the chicken breasts. Cover and refrigerate 2 to 4 hours.

Preheat oven to 375°F.

Place the baking pan in the oven and bake chicken for 45 minutes or until done, turning occasionally and basting. Remove bay leaves.

Serve hot.

Chicken Breast Apollo

Richard's daughter, Deborah, brought this recipe back from Greece. A few weeks after her return, on our wedding anniversary, we had attended a morning wedding and had enjoyed a Reward Meal brunch. Wanting to keep the evening a special celebration, Deborah made this dish for us as a surprise dinner, complete with mood music and candles. She is a gift we both enjoy.

³/₄ chopped cup chives

½ cup water

3 tablespoons fresh lemon juice

2½ tablespoons teriyaki sauce*

2 tablespoons olive oil

³/₄ teaspoon dried oregano

³/₄ teaspoon black pepper

4 large boneless, skinless chicken breast halves

In a medium bowl combine chives, water, lemon juice, teriyaki sauce, 1 tablespoon olive oil, oregano, and black pepper. Stir well.

Pour ¼ cup of the chive mixture into a 1-cup glass measure and set aside.

(continued on next page)

*Most recent Carbohydrate Addict's books may contain alternative guidelines for this ingredient. Consult your book's food lists for guidance. Use acceptable alternative as appropriate.

Put the remaining mixture and the chicken breasts into a large heavy-duty plastic zip-top bag. Marinate in refrigerator 20 minutes.

Preheat broiler.

Remove the chicken from the bag and discard the marinade.

Place the chicken in a shallow roasting pan that has been coated with the remaining 1 tablespoon olive oil.

Broil 7 minutes per side.

Remove chicken and let stand for 10 minutes.

Carve diagonally across the grain into thin slices. Set aside, and keep warm.

In a small skillet over high heat, heat the reserved ¼ cup of the chive mixture thoroughly, about 1 minute.

Pour over the chicken slices and serve immediately.

Michele's Broiled Turkey Patties

This is the favorite dish of an old friend with whom we have lost contact but often remember with gratitude.

2 tablespoons olive oil	1 teaspoon teriyaki sauce* or prepared mustard
½ cup finely chopped green bell pepper	½ teaspoon minced garlic
⅓ cup finely chopped celery	¼ teaspoon salt
1 pound ground turkey	¼ teaspoon pepper
2 medium eggs	

Coat a small nonstick skillet with 1 tablespoon of olive oil and place over medium heat.

Add green pepper and celery and sauté 4 to 5 minutes. Let cool.

In a medium bowl, combine sautéed mixture with turkey, eggs, teriyaki sauce (or mustard), garlic, salt, and pepper.

Preheat broiler.

Divide mixture into 4 equal portions, shaping each into a 4-inch patty.

Line a broiler pan with aluminum foil and coat the foil with the remaining 1 tablespoon olive oil.

Place the patties on the pan and broil 4 to 6 minutes per side, until thoroughly cooked.

*Most recent Carbohydrate Addict's books contain alternative guidelines for this ingredient. Consult your book's food lists for guidance. Use acceptable alternative as appropriate.

Peppery Chicken Salad

Sometimes we just want something that will perk up our taste buds. When you feel like that, too, this should do the trick!

1 cup sour cream

2 tablespoons lemon juice

1/2 teaspoon ground coriander

1/4 teaspoon salt

1/4 teaspoon crushed red pepper

1/4 teaspoon black pepper

3 cups boneless, skinless chicken breasts, cooked and chopped

1 green bell pepper, cut into thin strips

1/4 cup chopped red onion

1/4 cup chopped fresh parsley

2 1/4 ounces pitted olives, drained and sliced

In a medium bowl, combine sour cream, lemon juice, coriander, salt, crushed red pepper, and black pepper. Blend well.

Add chicken, green pepper, onion, parsley, and olives.

Toss and serve.

Classic Roasted Chicken

Rachael's mother was an excellent cook. She passed away at a young age and Rachael did not get a chance to get the benefit of her mother's great culinary skill and knowledge. This recipe is a variation of one of her mom's standards recalled from memory and re-created with love.

1 3-pound roasting chicken	½ teaspoon dried oregano
1 tablespoon olive oil	¼ teaspoon salt
½ teaspoon dried basil	⅛ teaspoon pepper

Preheat oven to 450°F.

Remove and discard the giblets and neck from chicken. Carefully rinse chicken under cold water, then pat dry.

Place the chicken, breast side up, on roasting rack in a roasting pan.

Coat chicken with olive oil, then sprinkle with basil, oregano, salt, and pepper.

Insert meat thermometer into the meaty part of a thigh, making sure not to touch bone.

Add an inch or so of water to roasting pan, making sure that water does not touch chicken.

Roast for 30 minutes.

Reduce oven temperature to 400°F and continue to roast until thermometer registers 180°F, 30 to 45 minutes.

Remove chicken from the oven, rest 15 minutes before carving, and serve warm.

Country Baked Chicken

When we met, Rachael was very poor. Trying desperately to work her way through a challenging doctoral program, she lived in a single-room occupancy hotel with no kitchen and only a tiny, quarter-size refrigerator. We chipped in together and bought an inexpensive electric convection oven. This was part of our first victory meal—and it was delicious!

1   3-pound broiler chicken, cut into pieces, excess fat removed

2   tablespoons fresh lemon juice

$1/8$ teaspoon salt

$1/8$ teaspoon freshly ground black pepper

1   teaspoon chopped fresh thyme

1   teaspoon chopped fresh rosemary

3   teaspoons chopped fresh sage

Preheat the oven to 400°F.

Rinse the chicken and pat dry with paper towels.

Combine the lemon juice, salt, pepper, thyme, rosemary, and sage.

Brush chicken with the lemon juice mixture and place in a 9 × 13-inch baking pan.

Bake for 55 to 60 minutes.

Serve warm.

Chicken Wings with Spicy Mustard Topping

We love this recipe because it tastes like junk food but isn't.

1 tablespoon olive oil

1 tablespoon Dijon mustard

1 tablespoon mustard seeds

½ teaspoon crumbled dried rosemary

1 clove garlic, minced

2 tablespoons dry white wine

¼ cup chicken stock, homemade only (page 26), or water

dash salt

¼ teaspoon black pepper

1 pound chicken wings

In a small saucepan, whisk together the oil, mustard, mustard seeds, rosemary, garlic, wine, chicken stock (or water), salt, and pepper. Warm the mixture but do not bring to boil. Allow to cool.

Place chicken wings in a bowl, add liquid, cover, and marinate overnight in refrigerator.

Preheat oven to 350°F.

Place wings on aluminum foil–lined baking sheet.

Pour half the marinade over wings and bake for 20 minutes.

Turn wings and pour remaining marinade over them. Bake for 20 minutes more.

Hungarian Chicken Paprikash

Richard's mother was from Croatia, his father, from Hungary.
This recipe goes back at least four generations.

¼ cup olive oil	1½ tablespoons paprika, sweet or hot
2 cloves garlic, minced	
1 3-pound chicken, cut into pieces	1 green bell pepper, sliced into rings
salt to taste	½ pound mushroom caps
black pepper to taste	1 cup sour cream

Heat oil in a large saucepan over medium heat; add garlic and sauté about 3 minutes.

Remove pan from heat. Sprinkle chicken with salt and black pepper and add to pan with paprika and half of the green pepper.

Cover pan with a tight-fitting lid and cook over very low heat.

After 30 minutes of cooking, add mushrooms.

Continue cooking until chicken is tender, an additional 15 minutes or so.

For even cooking, turn chicken occasionally. If liquid begins to disappear, add a few spoonfuls of water to prevent sticking.

When chicken is thoroughly cooked, transfer to a heated platter, continuing to heat liquid over medium heat.

Scrape bottom of pan to loosen any burned-on bits. Add only enough water to achieve a thick, gravylike consistency.

Remove from heat. Stir in sour cream to form a smooth blend of pan liquid and sour cream.

Pour mixture over chicken and garnish with the remaining green pepper.

Serve immediately.

Christmas Hens

Rachael's friend Sandi always makes you feel special; she takes entertaining very seriously. Here's one of Sandi's holiday recipes that we think you'll enjoy.

¹/₂ teaspoon lemon zest	2 2-pound Cornish game hens, halved, backbone discarded
juice of ¹/₂ lemon	
1 cup water	salt to taste
1¹/₂ tablespoons dry white wine	pepper to taste
¹/₄ teaspoon ground cloves	

Combine lemon zest and juice, water, wine, and ground cloves.

Marinate hens in lemon-clove mixture in covered bowl or sealed plastic bag in refrigerator overnight, turning occasionally to coat all sides.

Preheat oven to 450°F.

Season hen halves generously with salt and pepper; place, skin side up, in shallow roasting pan.

Pour marinade evenly over hen halves. Roast 30 to 45 minutes or until thoroughly cooked.

Serve warm or cold in salad.

Aromatic Chicken Breasts

We smelled the flavor of this wonderful dish long before we tasted it. It's a special gift from a good friend (who is too shy to allow us to include her name).

4 large boneless, skinless chicken breast halves	1 tablespoon teriyaki sauce*
salt to taste	3 tablespoons chopped parsley
black pepper to taste	2 teaspoons Dijon mustard
2 tablespoons olive oil	
3 tablespoons chopped fresh chives	¼ cup chicken stock, homemade only (page 26), or water
1½ tablespoons fresh lemon juice	

Place chicken breasts between sheets of wax paper and pound gently with a mallet.

Sprinkle with salt and pepper.

Heat olive oil in a large skillet. Add chicken and cook approximately 6 minutes over medium-high heat.

Turn and cook for an additional 6 minutes. Although overcooking will dry chicken out, be certain chicken is fully cooked.

Transfer breasts to a warm serving platter.

Add remaining ingredients, except the stock, to skillet. Cook 15 seconds, stirring constantly. Stir in the stock, and continue stirring until sauce is smooth. Pour all of this over the chicken and serve immediately.

*Most recent Carbohydrate Addict's books may contain alternative guidelines for this ingredient. Consult your book's food lists for guidance. Use acceptable alternative as appropriate.

Crusty Chicken Strips

In New York City you can find Spanish Chinese restaurants—an unusual combination to some, but commonplace to New Yorkers. This dish is just one of the wonderful recipes that come from the blend of these two dynamic cultures. We can picture our favorite booth at our favorite little hideaway whenever we make this variation.

2 tablespoons white vinegar	salt to taste
1 teaspoon Dijon mustard	black pepper to taste
¼ cup olive oil	2 eggs, beaten
1½ pounds boneless, skinless chicken breast halves, cut into 1-inch strips	6 cups curly endive, rinsed and spun dry

In a medium bowl, combine vinegar, mustard, and 2 tablespoons olive oil. Set aside.

Sprinkle chicken with salt and pepper. Dip each strip in beaten egg.

Heat remaining 2 tablespoons olive oil in a large skillet over medium heat. Sauté chicken until golden, about 5 minutes.

Arrange a portion of endive on each plate and top with chicken strips.

Drizzle with dressing and serve immediately.

Chicken in Cream Sauce

SERVES 6

We used to drive a twenty-one hour pilgrimage from New York to Disney World twice a year. Our favorite restaurant stop, one hour south of Savannah, Georgia, serves up good and gracious southern dishes such as this.

¼ cup olive oil	1 teaspoon prepared mustard
2 large cloves garlic	½ cup heavy cream
6 boneless, skinless chicken breast halves	1½ teaspoons sour cream
1 teaspoon salt	2 teaspoons minced fresh parsley
½ teaspoon black pepper or to taste	½ cup chopped scallions
1 cup chicken stock, homemade only (page 26), or water	

Heat the olive oil in a small skillet.

Add the garlic and cook over medium-low heat until the garlic is golden brown, about 3 minutes.

Sprinkle chicken breasts with salt and pepper.

Add chicken to skillet and sauté, turning once, until lightly browned and cooked through, about 6 minutes each side. Add parsley and scallions. Sauté for 2 additional minutes. Remove from heat.

Remove chicken to heated platter and keep warm.

Remove the garlic with a slotted spoon, drain on paper towels, slice, and set aside.

Immediately add chicken stock (or water) to warm pan and drippings. Add mustard, heavy cream, and sour cream and stir.

Spoon a portion of sauce over each chicken breast, sprinkle with toasted garlic, and serve immediately.

Creamy, Crunchy Chicken

SERVES 4

While sharing a vacation rental, our friends purloined this recipe from our files and, when we weren't looking, served us their version of one of our favorite dishes. Now it's our turn; we can change it back and they won't find out until they read it here!

¼ cup water

1 cup sour cream

1 whole frying chicken, cut up

salt to taste

black pepper to taste

½ cup olive oil

2 cups chopped celery

½ pound mushrooms, chopped

1 clove garlic, minced

½ teaspoon ground allspice

½ cup chicken stock, homemade only (page 26), or water

1 egg yolk

2 tablespoons light cream

Combine water and sour cream; add chicken and marinate in refrigerator for 20 minutes.

Season with salt and pepper.

Drain chicken, reserving marinade. Heat olive oil in large skillet and brown chicken pieces; do not cook chicken through.

Add celery, mushrooms, garlic, and allspice.

Add chicken stock (or water) to reserved marinade and pour over the chicken.

Simmer 45 to 60 minutes until thoroughly cooked (no pink inside).

Lower heat.

Beat egg yolk with cream. Stir into chicken mixture and cook until sauce thickens slightly. Do not allow to boil.

Serve immediately.

Gingery Chicken

For many years, Ana was our student and valued research assistant. Now that she is a wife and mother and medical professional, she still brings her creativity and love to all that she does, including her cooking!

1 egg yolk	½ cup chicken stock, homemade only (page 26), or water
4 boneless, skinless chicken breast halves	
salt to taste	2 cloves garlic, crushed
black pepper to taste	¼ cup chopped gingerroot
paprika to taste	¼ teaspoon ground nutmeg

Preheat oven to 375°F.

Beat egg yolk until light. Dip chicken into beaten yolk.

Season chicken with salt, pepper, and paprika to form a crust. Place in shallow roasting pan.

Heat chicken stock (or water) and stir in garlic, ginger, and nutmeg.

Pour over chicken.

Bake for 45 to 60 minutes, basting every 15 minutes.

Crustless Chicken Pot Pie

One late afternoon, while we were working hard to finish up some research, Rachael got an unexpected craving for some chicken pot pie. We had already had that day's Reward Meal. Somebody must have been listening with a great deal of love because this treat appeared at her low-carb meal a little later that day. What a wonderful surprise!

3	tablespoons olive oil	1½	cups chicken stock, homemade only (page 26), or water
1½	pounds boneless, skinless chicken breasts, cut into 1-inch pieces	2	celery stalks, chopped
2	cloves garlic, minced	1	green bell pepper, chopped
¼	teaspoon salt	1	cup shredded Cheddar cheese
¼	teaspoon black pepper		
1	tablespoon dry white wine		

Heat olive oil in a large skillet over high heat. Add chicken pieces and brown.

Add garlic. Sauté until garlic is limp, about 3 minutes. Sprinkle with salt and pepper.

Cook 1 minute, then add wine and chicken stock (or water).

Cover and simmer, stirring occasionally until chicken is tender and cooked through, approximately 20 minutes.

Preheat oven to 425°F.

Blanch celery and green peppers, drain and discard liquid.

When chicken is done, drain off liquid, reserving ½ cup.

Combine chicken, reserved chicken liquid, and vegetables.

Pour into pie pan, sprinkle with Cheddar cheese and bake for 20 minutes.

Cornish Game Hen Supreme

Cornish hens have their own special flavor. We like to complement that taste with sautéed vegetables and herbs worthy of this special dish.

4	small Cornish game hens	8	ounces mushrooms, chopped
	salt to taste	1	garlic clove, minced
	pepper to taste	2	tablespoons minced fresh basil
³/₄	cup olive oil	1	teaspoon dried oregano
4	celery stalks, chopped	2	tablespoons minced fresh parsley
1	green bell pepper, chopped		

Preheat oven to 325°F.

Season hens inside and out with salt and pepper.

Stir ¹/₂ cup olive oil with celery, green pepper, mushrooms, garlic, and herbs to form stuffing mixture.

Divide the vegetable mix into 4 equal parts and stuff each bird.

Place birds in baking dish, breast side up. Drizzle with remaining ¹/₄ cup olive oil.

Bake for 1 hour, until hens are thoroughly done.

Raise oven temperature to 500°F and brown hens for 10 minutes.

Warm Chicken Spinach Delight

Rachael loves this meal because the flavor steeps through the chicken and the vegetables, and the sauce makes it taste so good.

½ pound fresh spinach, washed and stems removed

3 tablespoons olive oil

12 asparagus spears, diced

4 boneless, skinless chicken breast halves, cut into 1 by 3-inch strips

1 clove garlic, crushed

6 ounces mushrooms, sliced

1 cup sour cream

Preheat 350°F.

Steam spinach until wilted; drain and chop. Place in casserole dish, cover, and keep warm.

Heat 2 tablespoons of olive oil in large skillet and sauté asparagus over medium heat until asparagus is fully cooked, about 2 minutes.

Remove asparagus and place evenly on spinach in casserole dish. Continue to keep covered and warm.

Add 1 tablespoon of olive oil to skillet, add chicken strips and garlic, and brown.

Add mushrooms and sauté until all ingredients are tender and thoroughly cooked.

Remove from heat.

With slotted spoon, remove chicken and mushrooms to casserole dish and continue to keep covered and warm.

In a small bowl, whisk 1 tablespoon of cooled oil and browned bits from bottom of skillet with sour cream.

When well blended, continue to whisk while slowly adding remaining cooled oil and browned bits a little at a time.

Spread sour cream mixture over chicken, spinach, and asparagus casserole and bake for 30 minutes.

Serve immediately.

Chicken Cordon Bleu

Inspired by a wonderful dish served at the famous Russian restaurant in New York, we use pork instead of ham to avoid the possibility of added sugars and glutamates, but the flavor remains rich and full.

4 boneless, skinless chicken breast halves	$\frac{1}{2}$ cup diced mozzarella cheese
$\frac{1}{2}$ cup minced cooked pork	2 large eggs
	salt to taste
$\frac{1}{2}$ cup grated Cheddar cheese	black pepper to taste
	$\frac{1}{4}$ cup olive oil

One at a time, place breast halves between two sheets of wax paper and pound flat.

With your hands, combine minced pork, cheeses, and eggs.

Form the mixture into four rolls about 3 inches long.

Place a roll on each breast half and fold breast half around it; begin with one long side, then fold in short sides, then finishing with the other long side—like an envelope.

Press edges together and roll each piece as it is finished in a sheet of wax paper. Refrigerate for 1 hour.

Heat olive oil in a fryer or wok to 350°F.

Unwrap the chicken pieces and fry, two at a time, in hot oil about 15 minutes on each side until browned evenly, thoroughly cooked, and firm to the touch. Salt and pepper to taste.

Gingered Chicken

We stuck some gingerroot, straight from the health food store, into the ground and watered it often. It sprouted new shoots and grew like crazy. We thought we'd cut off fresh pieces as we needed it for cooking but we've never had the nerve to cut it, so we still go to the market every time we need ginger and just enjoy watching our ginger plant grow. We think it's about to blossom (it makes us feel like our baby is about to give birth)!

2 whole boneless, skinless chicken breasts	1 ½-inch piece gingerroot, minced
2 tablespoons teriyaki sauce*	2 cloves garlic, minced
2 tablespoons chicken stock, homemade only (page 26), or water	1 egg
	1 cup olive oil

Pat chicken dry with paper towels. Cut into strips ½ inch wide by 3 inches long.

Make a marinade of teriyaki sauce, chicken stock (or water), ginger, and garlic.

Place chicken in marinade and refrigerate for at least 1 hour, turning chicken after half an hour.

Remove chicken from marinade and discard marinade. Drain chicken on paper towels.

Beat egg slightly with ½ teaspoon water. Dip chicken in egg mixture.

Heat oil to 350°F.

Fry chicken pieces in batches one layer deep until thoroughly cooked, crisp, and golden brown. Be sure to let oil come back up to 350°F between batches.

Drain chicken on paper towels and serve at once.

---

*Most recent Carbohydrate Addict's books may contain alternative guidelines for this ingredient. Consult your book's food lists for guidance. Use acceptable alternative as appropriate.

Chicken à la King

We have a hard time believing we can enjoy meals like this and still have a Reward Meal to look forward to!

½ cup olive oil
¾ cup sour cream
2 egg yolks,* beaten
½ cup chopped cauliflower
1 cup mushrooms, sliced
¼ cup chopped, blanched green bell pepper

3 cups cubed cooked chicken
1 tablespoon dry sherry
salt to taste
black pepper to taste
paprika to taste

Place olive oil in top of double boiler. Add sour cream. Heat over boiling water.

Remove from heat and add beaten egg yolks, cauliflower, mushrooms, green pepper, and chicken.

Season with dry sherry, salt, pepper, and paprika to taste.

*Use certified salmonella-free eggs only.

Baked Chicken Breasts with Mustard & Tarragon

Even though it's almost as easy to make this dish as plain baked chicken, many people aren't used to spending the tiny bit of energy it takes to make this sumptuous meal. Sometimes we have to be encouraged to take care of ourselves so, please, treat yourself like an honored guest!

4 boneless, skinless chicken breast halves	½ teaspoon black pepper
2 large cloves garlic, minced	1 large egg
	3 tablespoons Dijon mustard
1 tablespoon dried parsley	¼ cup olive oil
1 tablespoon dried tarragon	parsley sprigs
1 teaspoon salt	2 tablespoons capers

One at a time, place chicken breasts between two pieces of wax paper and pound gently to even thickness.

In shallow dish, mix together garlic, parsley, tarragon, salt, and pepper.

In another dish, beat egg with mustard.

Dip each chicken breast into the beaten egg mixture and then in the garlic/herb mixture to coat evenly. Place on a baking sheet, cover with wax paper, and refrigerate for several hours.

Heat oil in a large nonstick frying pan and, over medium-high heat, brown chicken well on both sides. Continue cooking over low-medium heat until chicken is cooked through, about 7 minutes per side.

Transfer to serving plates; garnish each with parsley sprig and capers.

Island Lime Chicken

As she grew older, we had Richard's mom living in the apartment next door to us. We could see her all of the time and, thanks to our good friend and apartment house owner, Sy, we could afford to keep her with us. Mom's generous Haitian caretaker made sumptuous dishes such as this for Mom and often made "extra" so that we would have a warm and wonderful dinner waiting for us after a hard day of teaching and research at the medical school.

$^1/_2$ cup fresh lime juice	salt to taste
6 tablespoons olive oil	black pepper to taste
8 chicken pieces, with skin and bone	3 ounces mushroom caps, sliced

Preheat broiler.

In small bowl, mix lime juice and 2 tablespoons of olive oil.

One piece at a time, dip chicken in mixture to coat each piece completely.

On foil-lined baking pan, arrange chicken in single layer and sprinkle with salt and pepper.

Arrange broiler rack at least 6 inches from heat.

Broil chicken 12 to 15 minutes, then turn and pour remaining coating mixture over chicken.

Broil another 12 to 15 minutes more, or until fork can be inserted in chicken with ease.

While the chicken cooks, place remaining 4 tablespoons olive oil and the mushrooms in a medium skillet and sauté over medium-high heat for 5 minutes.

Set aside.

When the chicken is done, pour mushrooms and oil over chicken and return to oven for about 2 minutes or until mushrooms are hot.

Chicken Breasts with Pepper Sauce

SERVES 4

We love to serve this dish with a crisp green salad. The tastes balance and enhance each other.

2 tablespoons minced garlic	1/2 cup half-and-half
4 boneless, skinless chicken breast halves	1/4 cup sour cream
1 to 2 tablespoons olive oil	1 tablespoon green peppercorns
1/4 cup dry white wine	1 teaspoon dried basil

Preheat oven to 400°F.

In a large skillet over medium-high heat, sauté garlic and chicken breasts in olive oil until chicken is lightly browned on both sides. Add wine and cook for an additional 5 minutes.

Transfer to a baking dish with sauce and bake for 12 to 15 minutes.

While the chicken is baking, use the same skillet over medium heat to heat the half-and-half, sour cream, peppercorns, and basil, stirring constantly until the sauce coats the back of a spoon. Do not boil.

Spoon the sauce over each piece of baked chicken and serve.

Hot and Crispy Chicken Halves

You can use the flavorful sauce in this dish on any poultry or fish. It's great on chicken, as we serve it here, but we think you'll branch out to quickly to include it with other proteins, as well.

2 small whole chickens, halved

2 tablespoons olive oil

3 tablespoons lemon juice

2 teaspoons salt

1 teaspoon dried tarragon

1 teaspoon paprika

$1/2$ teaspoon hot pepper sauce

Preheat oven to 375°F.

Place chicken halves, skin side down, in a shallow nonstick baking pan.

In a small bowl, combine olive oil, lemon juice, salt, tarragon, paprika, and hot pepper sauce.

Brush about half of the mixture generously over the 4 chicken halves.

Bake 50 to 60 minutes. Turning chicken after the first 30 minutes.

Brush several times with remaining oil mixture during baking. Chicken is done when tender to the touch of a fork.

Saucy Turkey Breast

We all know turkey isn't only for Thanksgiving anymore, but we sometimes forget to think of it as a choice for a tasty, low-carbohydrate meal. Here's a whole new take on good old turkey.

2 tablespoons olive oil	¹/₂ cup sour cream
1¹/₄ pounds home-cooked turkey breast—broiled, roasted, or baked and sliced	2 teaspoons prepared mustard
¹/₂ cup heavy cream	¹/₄ tablespoons capers, drained

Heat 1 tablespoon of oil in each of two large skillets. Sauté turkey slices over medium-high heat 1 to 2 minutes per side, then remove to a warmed plate. Cover plate with foil to keep warm.

In a medium pan over medium-high heat, warm heavy cream, stirring frequently, until it begins to bubble.

Stir in sour cream, mustard, capers, and any turkey juices that have collected on the plate.

Bring sauce to boiling point, stirring constantly.

Spoon sauce over turkey slices and serve immediately.

142 ❖ The Carbohydrate Addict's Cookbook

Western-Style Roasted Chicken and Green Peppers

Originally, this dish was called Pollo de Oro *which, roughly translated means "Chicken of Gold." We've also seen it called* Pollo Verde *("Green Chicken"). While the restaurants battle out the "correct" name, we just cook up this version and enjoy it!*

3 tablespoons olive oil	1 teaspoon crushed sage
1 3-pound roasting chicken, skinned	6 tablespoons white vinegar
2 large cloves garlic	3 green bell peppers, cleaned and halved
1 tablespoon fresh tarragon, minced	

Preheat oven to 350°F.

Place chicken in roasting rack in baking pan, breast side up.

Peel and halve garlic cloves and rub surface of chicken with cut garlic. Then place the garlic cloves inside chicken.

In a small bowl, combine olive oil, tarragon, sage, and vinegar.

Pour over surface of chicken and inside cavity.

Place green peppers below chicken in 1 to 1½ inches water (water should not touch chicken).

Roast 60 minutes (until juice runs clear when a sharp knife is inserted in thigh of bird), basting every 15 minutes.

Slice or cut into serving pieces and serve with green peppers and cooking liquid.

Curried-Basil Chicken

One of the keys to success in Indian cooking is not to overdo the curry powder. Taste it on the first making and decide on the right amount of curry powder to suit your tastes.

2	tablespoons olive oil	$1/3$	cup heavy cream
4	large boneless, skinless chicken breast halves	$1^1/2$	teaspoons curry powder
	salt to taste	2	tablespoons dried basil
	black pepper to taste	8	medium romaine lettuce leaves, rinsed and dried
1	clove garlic, chopped		

Heat olive oil in a large frying pan over medium-high heat.

Sprinkle chicken with salt and pepper and cook about 4 minutes, turning occasionally.

Add garlic and continue cooking for 30 seconds.

Stir in $1/4$ cup of the cream and 2 tablespoons water. Reduce heat to medium, cover, and simmer about 10 minutes, until chicken is cooked through.

Transfer chicken to a serving plate and keep warm.

Whisk in remaining cream and curry powder and bring to a simmer.

Add basil. Season to taste with salt and pepper.

Place chicken pieces on romaine lettuce leaves. Pour sauce over the chicken breasts and serve.

Stuffed Chicken Breasts

We were about to go on vacation and Richard wanted to use up all the leftovers in the refrigerator. After eating this dish, we knew we'd miss our home cooking all the more while we were away.

½ pound fresh spinach	black pepper to taste
4 tablespoons olive oil	4 large boneless, skinless chicken breast halves
1 tablespoon chopped onion	
½ pound mushrooms, chopped	2 tablespoons dry white wine
1 clove garlic, crushed	fresh parsley, chopped
½ teaspoon dried oregano	lemon wedges

Wash spinach, place in saucepan, and cook, covered only with the water clinging to the leaves, until barely wilted. Drain spinach well, squeezing out excess water. Chop and set aside.

Heat 2 tablespoons oil in a skillet until hot; add onion and mushrooms and sauté until tender.

Add garlic, oregano, spinach, and pepper to taste.

Cook and stir for 1 minute. Set aside.

Meanwhile, place each chicken breast between two layers of wax paper and pound with rolling pin or heavy plate edge until about ¼ inch thick.

Preheat oven to 350°F.

Spoon a quarter of the mushroom and spinach mixture onto center of each chicken breast; roll lengthwise and secure with wooden toothpicks. Place rolls in a 9-inch shallow baking pan.

Combine wine with remaining 2 tablespoons oil and spoon over chicken. Bake, uncovered, until chicken is tender, about 55 minutes. Baste often.

Sprinkle with chopped parsley and serve with lemon wedges.

Barbecued Lemon Chicken

SERVES 8

When people ask us for a low-carb substitute for barbecue sauce we give them this recipe. Later, many have written back to say they like it so much, they enjoy this dish at Reward Meals as well.

2 whole chickens, cut into pieces	1 teaspoon salt
1 cup olive oil	1 teaspoon paprika
1/2 cup lemon juice	2 teaspoons onion powder
1 teaspoon teriyaki sauce*	1/2 teaspoon dried thyme
	1/2 teaspoon garlic powder

Place chicken into shallow dish or pan. Combine all other ingredients and pour over chicken. Cover dish with foil; refrigerate overnight.

Prepare grill.

Place chicken on hot grill for 25 minutes; then turn and cook 25 minutes more until chicken is thoroughly cooked.

*Most recent Carbohydrate Addict's books may contain alternative guidelines for this ingredient. Consult your book's food lists for guidance. Use acceptable alternative as appropriate.

Cabbage Rolls with Turkey-Cheese Stuffing

SERVES 4 TO 6

One of the few times that Rachael had a bad head cold, we made this to tempt her taste buds. It's been tempting us, and satisfying us as well, ever since.

1 head savoy cabbage	1 teaspoon chopped fresh parsley
1 pound ground turkey	
1 egg	salt to taste
½ cup chicken stock, homemade only (page 26), or water	black pepper to taste
	1½ cups diced mozzarella cheese
1 teaspoon sage, crumbled	6 bacon slices*

Remove twelve large leaves of cabbage and cut out tough inner part of rib.

Blanch each leaf 1 minute until pliable.

Combine ground turkey, egg, 2 tablespoons stock (or water), sage, and parsley.

Add salt and pepper to taste.

Preheat oven to 350°F.

Divide turkey mixture into twelve parts, and form into 4-inch ovals.

Divide mozzarella cheese into twelve parts. Place a turkey oval and some mozzarella at stem end of each cabbage leaf, fold in sides, and roll up.

Place rolls in one layer in shallow baking dish.

Pour remaining 6 tablespoons stock (or water) over all.

Precook bacon until lightly done. Place half a slice on each roll.

Bake for 30 minutes, basting twice, until turkey is thoroughly cooked.

---

*Most recent Carbohydrate Addict's books may contain alternative guidelines for this ingredient. Consult your book's food lists for guidance. Use acceptable alternative as appropriate.

SEAFOOD

From Block Island, Rhode Island, to Kangaroo Island, Australia; from Grand Cayman Island to Oahu, Hawaii, we mark our travels by the luscious seafood meals we remember.

These are the meals of our lives, moments of pleasure we share with each other, for the first time to be enjoyed without fear, embarrassment, or self-blame.

God gave us the ability to enjoy the food that nourishes us and to appreciate the beauty and sanctity from which it comes.

Classic Shrimp Scampi

SERVES 6

*Richard makes this as a special treat—just for the two of us—
when we want something that reminds us to put ourselves first!*

36 large shrimp	$1/4$ cup minced fresh parsley
3 tablespoons olive oil	$1/4$ cup fresh lemon juice
1 cup minced green bell pepper	$1/2$ teaspoon salt
8 cloves garlic, crushed	$1/4$ teaspoon pepper
$1/2$ cup dry white wine, or chicken stock, homemade only, (page 26)	paprika

Leaving the tails intact, peel the shrimp.

Starting at tail end of each shrimp, butterfly underside, cutting to, but not through, the back of shrimp.

Arrange 6 shrimp, cut side up, in each of 6 gratin dishes and set aside.

Preheat broiler.

Heat olive oil in a small skillet over medium heat.

Add green pepper and garlic and sauté 2 to 3 minutes.

Remove from heat; stir in wine (or stock), parsley, lemon juice, salt, and pepper.

Pour the mixture evenly over each serving, sprinkle paprika on shrimp, and broil 6 to 8 minutes.

Serve warm on spinach leaves or bed of lettuce.

Barnacle Bill's Scallops

Amid the hustle and the bustle of the Esplanade in Cairns, Australia, Barnacle Bill's is our favorite seafood restaurant. We can eat there night after night and always enjoy it. When we're thousands of miles away from there, this dish is the next best thing.

⅓ cup fresh lime juice	1 teaspoon chopped fresh jalapeño pepper, or dried equivalent
¼ cup minced fresh parsley	
¼ cup chopped green bell pepper	½ teaspoon dried cilantro
	salt to taste
¼ cup chopped scallion	1½ pounds sea scallops, rinsed and drained
1 tablespoon olive oil	
1 clove garlic, minced	4 tablespoons grated Parmesan cheese

Preheat broiler.

In a medium bowl combine all ingredients and stir well.

Divide mixture evenly among 4 ovenproof dishes.

Place dishes on a baking sheet and broil 8 to 10 minutes.

Serve immediately.

Horseradish Scallops and Asparagus

Near Disneyland Paris, there's a little restaurant with blue and white checkered tablecloths. They serve this dish and only one or two other choices. They believe that less is more. We agree.

1½ pounds sea scallops, rinsed and drained	12 spears asparagus, woody stems cut off, sliced in diagonal pieces
3 tablespoons prepared white horseradish	1 tablespoon chopped fresh chives
3 tablespoons olive oil	

In a medium bowl, combine scallops and horseradish and toss well. Marinate for 1 hour in refrigerator.

Heat olive oil in a nonstick skillet over medium-high heat.

Remove the scallops from the marinade and reserve horseradish marinade.

Add half the scallops to the skillet and cook about 1 minute per side until cooked through.

Remove scallops to a plate and keep warm. Repeat with the remaining scallops.

In the same pan used for the scallops, cook the asparagus for 3 minutes over medium-high heat, shaking the pan constantly. Remove the asparagus to the plate with the scallops.

Using the same skillet over a high heat, warm the reserved horseradish marinade, about 3 minutes.

Return the scallops and asparagus to the skillet and coat well with the contents of the skillet.

Sprinkle with chives and serve immediately.

Block Island Shrimp

Our lawn was the setting for the yearly square dance at our home on the little island twelve miles into the Atlantic. Everyone brought something special for the potluck dinner that always followed. The maker of this dish would have been invited on the strength of her good cooking alone. She loves our version even more than the original.

1 pound jumbo shrimp
¼ cup olive oil
1 tablespoon minced garlic
1 tablespoon chopped fresh rosemary
1 tablespoon chopped fresh thyme

½ teaspoon freshly ground black pepper
cayenne pepper to taste
¼ teaspoon salt
3 eggs, beaten well

Peel and devein the shrimp, leaving the tails intact. Pat dry and put aside.

Combine the garlic, rosemary, thyme, black pepper, cayenne pepper, and salt.

Dip shrimp in egg and dredge in dry mixture.

Fry in olive oil for 4 to 8 minutes, turning once.

Savory Fish with Vegetables

There's a store on Block Island, Rhode Island, that sells fish that has been been caught that day. You've never tasted better fish in your life. Each piece of fish comes with a free recipe and a quotation to inspire. The quotation failed to make it but the recipe inspired this dish.

1½ cups diced green bell peppers

3 leeks, cut into 2-inch julienne

1 celery stalk, cut into 2-inch julienne

2 pounds fish fillets of choice, cleaned and halved

2 cups fish stock, homemade only (see variation, page 26), or water

2 tablespoons teriyaki sauce*

2 teaspoons lemon juice

1 cup heavy cream

  salt to taste

  black pepper to taste

12 large romaine lettuce or spinach leaves

Preheat oven to 450°F.

Cook green peppers, leeks, and celery in boiling, lightly salted water for 30 seconds.

Drain and refresh in cold water.

Put fish, 1 cup of the fish stock (or water), and teriyaki sauce in a roasting pan large enough to hold the fish fillets.

(continued on next page)

---

*Most recent Carbohydrate Addict's books may contain alternative guidelines for this ingredient. Consult your book's food lists for guidance. Use acceptable alternative as appropriate.

Sprinkle with 1 tablespoon of lemon juice and the cooked vegetables. Cover lightly with foil, put into oven, and immediately turn heat down to 350°F.

Braise for 10 to 12 minutes, basting every few minutes with juices from bottom of pan.

The fish is done when it flakes with a fork.

With spatulas, remove fish to a large serving platter. Cover with foil to keep warm.

Over medium-high heat in a medium-size saucepan, simmer remaining 1 cup fish stock, about 10 minutes, until reduced by half.

Add cream and cook an additional 8 to 10 minutes, until the sauce is reduced by a third.

Season well with salt, pepper, and remaining 1 tablespoon lemon juice.

Place two romaine lettuce or spinach leaves on each plate and fill with equal portions of fish and vegetables.

Tuna Steak Supreme

We love to serve this dish to guests who think they don't like fish.
They invariably end up asking for the recipe!

4 tablespoons olive oil	salt to taste
2 cloves garlic, minced	black pepper to taste
3 cups spinach leaves, washed, patted dry, and chopped	¼ cup grated Parmesan cheese
2 pounds boneless, skinless tuna steaks	

Preheat oven to 450°F.

Heat 2 tablespoons of olive oil in a small skillet over medium heat.

Add garlic and stir for 2 minutes.

Add spinach leaves and stir to coat. Set aside.

Line a baking sheet with foil. Spread remaining 2 tablespoons olive oil over the center of the foil and lay tuna steaks on the oiled surface.

Season steaks with salt and pepper.

Sprinkle each steak with Parmesan cheese and bake 6 minutes.

Turn each steak. Top each with a portion of the garlic, oil, spinach mixture. Bake for 5 more minutes until thoroughly cooked.

Serve immediately.

156 ❖ The Carbohydrate Addict's Cookbook

Saucy Broiled Sole Fillets

The green sauce makes this dish very special. Richard invented it on St. Patrick's Day, saying that if we dripped anything on our clothes, at least we'd look like we were dressed for the holiday. Gotta love him!

4 large sole fillets	2 cups sliced mushrooms
3 tablespoons olive oil	2 teaspoons minced garlic
1 green bell pepper, chopped	1 teaspoon lemon juice
	1/4 teaspoon teriyaki sauce*

Preheat broiler.

Wash fillets and pat dry.

In a small skillet over medium-high heat, sauté the green pepper and mushrooms in 2 tablespoons of olive oil.

Drain off the oil and place the sautéed vegetables in food processor.

Add garlic, lemon juice, and teriyaki sauce.

Purée until thick spread is formed.

Spoon mixture into a small bowl, and refrigerate for 2 hours.

Use 1 tablespoon olive oil to coat a large baking sheet.

Place fish fillets on oiled baking sheet. Spread approximately 1 tablespoon of green pepper mixture onto each fish fillet.

Broil for 5 minutes. Turn filets and spread with green pepper mixture as before. Return to oven. Cook 5 more minutes. The fish is done when it flakes with a fork.

Serve with any remaining green pepper sauce.

*Most recent Carbohydrate Addict's books may contain alternative guidelines for this ingredient. Consult your book's food lists for guidance. Use acceptable alternative as appropriate.

Monkfish in Parchment

SERVES 4

Rachael loves this dish. The parchment seals in all of the juices and flavor.

2 tablespoons olive oil	2 teaspoons minced fresh chives
1½ pounds monkfish	
2 tablespoons teriyaki sauce*	2 teaspoons minced fresh parsley
⅓ cup green minced onions	
juice of 1 lemon	¼ cup dry white wine

Preheat oven to 400°F.

Coat a 9 by 12-inch baking dish with the olive oil.

Arrange 4 large sheets of parchment paper on a table or counter.

Cut monkfish into 4 equal parts and lay each piece on a sheet of parchment.

Sprinkle with teriyaki sauce, green onions, lemon juice, chives, parsley, and wine.

Crimp edges of parchment together and roll to seal on all sides. Place parchment packets seam side down on baking sheet.

Bake for 20 minutes.

When ready to serve, unroll parchment packets and place fish on platter.

Spoon cooking liquid and herbs over top and serve.

*Most recent Carbohydrate Addict's books may contain alternative guidelines for this ingredient. Consult your book's food lists for guidance. Use acceptable alternative as appropriate.

Broiled Swordfish with Cilantro Oil

SERVES 4

The flavorful sauce that we discovered on Grand Cayman Island, British West Indies, brings a whole new taste to any fish.

4 medium center-cut swordfish steaks

¼ cup olive oil

1 bunch cilantro, washed, stems removed

juice of ¼ lemon

salt to taste

black pepper to taste

Preheat broiler.

Lightly coat steaks with 2 tablespoons olive oil and place fish on oiled, aluminum foil–lined broiling pan.

Broil 3 to 4 minutes per side. Fillets should be firm to the touch with a fork when cooked long enough.

While steaks broil, place cilantro, remaining 2 tablespoons olive oil, and lemon juice into a blender and mix for 5 to 10 seconds. Season with salt and pepper.

Serve steaks warm with a portion of cilantro mixture over each piece.

Mixed Seafood Salad

This is an herbal "everything-but-the-kitchen sink" recipe and we really enjoy the unusual blend of flavors. As with their vegetables, most people overcook seafood. The secret is to cook it just until it's done and stop before it loses its sweet flavor and tender texture.

1 large green bell pepper	1½ tablespoons fresh lemon juice
¼ cup dry white wine, or chicken stock, home-made only (page 26)	1½ teaspoons olive oil
	¼ teaspoon salt
16 fresh clams, scrubbed	⅛ teaspoon dried rosemary, crushed
16 fresh mussels, scrubbed	⅛ teaspoon pepper
¼ pound shrimp, peeled and deveined	4 medium pitted ripe olives, halved
2 tablespoons chopped fresh parsley	4 pitted green olives, halved
	1 clove garlic, crushed

Preheat broiler.

Cut bell pepper in half lengthwise; discard the seeds and membranes.

Place pepper, skin side up, on a foil-covered baking sheet, then flatten with your hand.

Broil 8 to 10 minutes, until blackened.

Place the pepper in a heavy-duty zip-top plastic bag, seal and let stand 15 minutes. Peel pepper and cut into julienne strips. Set aside.

(continued on next page)

In a large skillet over high heat, bring wine (or stock) to a boil. Add clams, mussels, and shrimp. Reduce heat, cover, and simmer 4 to 5 minutes. Discard any unopened shells.

Remove the contents of the skillet with a slotted spoon, and set aside.

Discard all but 1 tablespoon of the remaining liquid. Remove meat from 12 clam and 12 mussel shells and discard the shells. Set aside remaining 4 clams and 4 mussels in their shells.

Cut the shrimp in half lengthwise and place in a large bowl. Add shelled clams, mussels, shrimp, reserved cooking liquid, bell pepper, parsley, lemon juice, olive oil, salt, rosemary, pepper, olives, and garlic.

Toss everything well.

Cover and refrigerate 2 to 3 hours.

Decorate with whole clams and mussels in shells. Serve cold.

Salmon Patties

Rachael invented this recipe one Saturday afternoon when she was hungry for her mother's old-fashioned salmon croquettes, but with a low-carb twist.

2	6½-ounce cans salmon, drained	1 tablespoon lemon juice
3	tablespoons chopped fresh parsley	1 teaspoon teriyaki sauce*
		¼ teaspoon salt
		black pepper to taste
1	clove garlic, minced	2 eggs

Preheat oven to 350°F.

Remove skin and bones from canned salmon, and flake salmon.

Add parsley, garlic, lemon juice, teriyaki sauce, salt, pepper, and eggs. Blend well.

Form into 4 patties and place in oiled baking pan.

Bake for 20 to 25 minutes and serve warm.

*Most recent Carbohydrate Addict's books may contain alternative guidelines for this ingredient. Consult your book's food lists for guidance. Use alternative seasoning as appropriate.

Baked Salmon with Herbs

This dish costs a fortune at one of this country's most expensive restaurants. This variation costs a whole lot less but tastes just as good—even better, we think!

2 tablespoons dried basil	1½ tablespoons white vinegar
1½ ounces fresh gingerroot, peeled	salt to taste
	black pepper to taste
3 large cloves garlic, peeled	4 tablespoons sesame oil
1 small chile pepper, chopped	6 large salmon fillets

Put basil, gingerroot, garlic, chili pepper, vinegar, salt, pepper, and 3 tablespoons sesame oil into a food processor and process to a smooth paste.

Brush salmon fillets with remaining 1 tablespoon sesame oil, then transfer, skin side down, to a baking dish. Spread 2 tablespoons of the paste on each fillet. Cover and refrigerate 2 hours.

Preheat oven to 400°F.

Bake salmon fillets about 12 minutes. The fish is done when it flakes with a fork. Serve immediately.

Steamed Mussels Peppercorn

*In six months' time, Rachael's brand-new fishing pole never
yielded a single fish. One day at the beach on Block Island,
Rhode Island, while still trying to catch her first one, we hooked
a floating mass of mussels and pulled it in. We abandoned our
fishing for that day, grabbed our unexpected bounty from the sea,
and headed for home.*

18 mussels, scrubbed well	10 whole peppercorns
1 tablespoon chopped onion	1/2 teaspoon chopped fresh parsley
1 clove garlic, chopped	1 cup water
1 tablespoon chopped celery	2 tablespoons olive oil
1/4 teaspoon dried thyme	

Place mussels in basket of steamer.

In steamer of large pot filled with 2 inches of water,
combine the remaining ingredients and steam over high
heat until shells open.

Remove mussels to warm plate, discarding any that
have not opened, and serve.

Parmesan Shrimp

Shrimp scampi, shrimp cocktail, or fried shrimp—shrimp is wonderful seafood that can be prepared in a great many equally delicious ways. This is one of our favorites and Richard's daughter, Caroline, loves to surprise us with this treat.

1½ pounds shrimp, peeled and deveined

¼ cup olive oil

½ pound mushrooms, sliced

1½ cups sour cream

1 tablespoon chopped chives

½ tablespoon fresh chopped parsley

salt to taste

black pepper to taste

½ teaspoon paprika

¼ cup grated Parmesan cheese

½ cup finely diced celery

Preheat broiler.
In a large skillet over medium heat, sauté shrimp in olive oil for 3 minutes.

Add mushrooms and sauté until tender.
Blend in sour cream, chives, and parsley.
Season with salt, pepper, and paprika.
Cook 5 minutes, stirring continuously.
Spoon into 4 ovenproof serving dishes, sprinkle tops with Parmesan cheese and broil for 3 to 5 minutes until tops are golden.
Sprinkle each dish with chopped celery and serve hot.

Bounty of the Sea

SERVES 4 TO 6

The cost of this recipe is pretty high; the ingredients don't come cheap. But when we want something special for ourselves or something extraordinary for guests, it can't be beat.

½ pound mushrooms, sliced	paprika to taste
½ cup chopped scallions	½ pound cooked crabmeat
6 tablespoons olive oil	½ cup cooked lobster meat
¾ cup heavy cream	12 large cooked shrimp
salt to taste	¼ cup grated Parmesan
black pepper to taste	cheese

Preheat oven to 450°F.

In a medium skillet, sauté mushrooms and scallions in olive oil for 5 minutes.

Add cream and bring to a boil, stirring constantly. Remove from heat and season with salt, pepper, and paprika.

Place crabmeat, lobster meat, and shrimp in a shallow oiled casserole dish.

Cover with the mushroom cream sauce and sprinkle with cheese. Bake for 10 minutes, then brown under broiler for 2 to 3 minutes.

Blackened Fish Fillets

On a steep hill in San Francisco, there's a restaurant where the whole dining room is sloped. It's strange walking to your table and odd to look around the room but dishes such as this make it worth the experience.

1 tablespoon paprika	$^1/_2$ teaspoon dried thyme
$^3/_4$ teaspoon cayenne pepper	$^1/_2$ teaspoon dried oregano
1 teaspoon salt	dash cumin
$^1/_2$ teaspoon black pepper	$^3/_4$ cup olive oil
$^1/_2$ teaspoon white pepper	2 pounds fish fillets, $^1/_2$ to
1 teaspoon onion powder	$^3/_4$ inch thick
1 teaspoon garlic powder	

Mix spices and herbs together on large plate.

Place 3 tablespoons of olive oil in heavy skillet. Place remaining 9 tablespoons olive oil in a 9 by 12 by 1-inch pan.

Turn heat under skillet to high. Quickly dip each fillet in the olive oil in the pan and then dip in the spice mixture, patting the fillets by hand.

Cook fish on each side for 2 to 3 minutes, being careful when turning the fillets over. The fish will look charred—"blackened"—and there may be some smoke, but there should not be an excessive amount.

The blackening forms a spicy, crunchy coating, sealing in moisture and flavor.

Serve warm.

West Indian Scallops

On Grand Cayman Island, we have enjoyed some of the best scuba diving in the world. Restaurants abound with so many "island originals" that it's hard to choose just one. Here's our homemade version of one the most outstanding we have found.

2 tablespoons olive oil	$^1/_2$ teaspoon cumin seed
$1^1/_2$ pounds sea scallops, rinsed and drained	$^1/_4$ teaspoon saffron
1 teaspoon dried chervil	$^1/_2$ cup grated Parmesan cheese
$^1/_2$ teaspoon dried marjoram	$^1/_2$ cup capers
$^1/_2$ teaspoon dried thyme	

Preheat broiler.

In an oven-safe skillet, heat olive oil until it smokes but does not burn.

Quickly sauté scallops for about 3 to 4 minutes until completely opaque and cooked through.

Stir in herbs.

Sprinkle with Parmesan cheese and place under broiler until lightly browned.

Top with capers and serve.

Baked Flounder

We find that the addition of sour cream and allspice makes a tried-and-true favorite into a dish that's very special.

3 pounds flounder fillets	¹/₄ teaspoon peppercorns
¹/₄ cup white vinegar	¹/₄ teaspoon ground allspice
1 teaspoon garlic powder	¹/₂ cup sour cream

Place flounder fillets, skin side up, in a shallow ceramic, glass, or enameled baking dish.

Combine vinegar, garlic powder, peppercorns, and all-spice and pour over fish.

Marinate in the refrigerator for 1 hour.

Pour off marinade.

Preheat oven to 350°F.

Turn fish skin side down and spread top with sour cream. Bake for 20 to 25 minutes, until fish flakes easily with a fork.

Baked Tuna Steak

SERVES 4

We can count on this friendly favorite to deliver a satisfying meal every time.

1 teaspoon salt
¼ teaspoon black pepper
2 cloves garlic, minced
¼ teaspoon red pepper flakes
4 small tuna steaks

½ cup olive oil
¼ cup lemon juice
2 tablespoons teriyaki sauce*

Preheat oven to 375°F.

Combine salt, pepper, garlic, and pepper flakes together thoroughly and rub on both sides of tuna steaks.

Place 2 tablespoons of olive oil in shallow baking dish and lay in the tuna steaks.

Combine remaining 6 tablespoons olive oil, lemon juice, and teriyaki sauce and pour over fish. Bake for 30 minutes or until fish flakes easily with a fork. Baste with seasoned oil mixture 2 or 3 times during baking.

*Most recent Carbohydrate Addict's books may contain alternative guidelines for this ingredient. Consult your book's food lists for guidance. Use acceptable alternative as appropriate.

Baked Herby Shrimp

We usually make extra servings of this recipe so that we can enjoy the leftovers cold, either as a second meal or as an appetizer.

3/4 cup olive oil

1 clove garlic, minced

1 teaspoon chopped fresh parsley

1 teaspoon chopped fresh chervil

1 teaspoon chopped fresh tarragon

1/8 teaspoon turmeric

1/8 teaspoon ground mace

1/8 teaspoon ground coriander

1 teaspoon salt

1 teaspoon dry sherry

1 1/2 pounds shrimp, cooked and peeled

Preheat oven to 450°F.

Combine 1/2 cup olive oil with garlic, herbs, spices, and salt.

Beat in sherry.

Fold in shrimp.

Place remaining 1/4 cup oil in a baking dish and add layers of shrimp.

Bake for 15 minutes.

Broiled Lobster Tails with a Twist

Among his many jobs, our friend Alvin is a lobster fisherman. When we lived on Block Island, he used to show up at our door with all the lobsters that the three of us could ever eat. Alvin could have hauled in a pretty penny for those lobsters, but he chose to share them with us instead. And did we have a celebration! Good food, good friends, all the time in the world to share it, and no guilt. Who could have asked for more? To this day, Alvin is as generous as he is gentle and caring.

4	large lobster tails		dash paprika
3	tablespoons olive oil	2	tablespoons dry white wine
2	tablespoons grated Parmesan cheese	2	tablespoons lemon juice
1½	teaspoons minced fresh parsley	1	clove garlic, crushed

Using kitchen shears, make a lengthwise cut through the top of the shell of each lobster tail.

Press the shell open and, starting at the cut end of the tail, carefully loosen the lobster meat from bottom of the shell.

(continued on next page)

Be careful to keep meat attached at the other end of the tail as you lift meat through the cut, and place on top of the cut shell.

Place lobster tails in a shallow roasting pan coated with 1 tablespoon of olive oil.

Preheat broiler.

In a small bowl, combine Parmesan cheese, parsley, paprika, and 1 tablespoon of olive oil. Set aside.

In another small bowl, combine remaining 1 tablespoon of olive oil, wine, lemon juice, and garlic; stir well.

Brush lobster with half of wine mixture.

Broil 9 to 10 minutes, or until lobster flesh turns opaque, basting with remaining wine mixture after 5 minutes.

Sprinkle Parmesan mixture evenly over lobster, and broil an additional 30 seconds.

Creamy Mussel Stew

The broth in which you cook your seafood can make all the difference to the end result. Add to the pot any good additional herbs that you enjoy.

18 mussels, scrubbed well
1 tablespoon chopped onion
1 clove garlic, chopped
1 tablespoon chopped celery
¼ teaspoon dried thyme
10 whole peppercorns
½ teaspoon chopped fresh parsley
2 cups water
2 tablespoons olive oil
½ cup sour cream
½ cup heavy cream
1 teaspoon prepared white horseradish

Place mussels in basket of steamer.

Combine all of the ingredients except last four items in bottom of steamer and steam the mussels over high heat until shells open.

Remove mussels to plate, discarding broth and any mussels that have not opened.

Heat oil in medium skillet over medium flame.

One at a time, slowly add the sour cream, heavy cream, and horseradish, stirring until smooth.

As creamy mixture begins to boil, add mussels, stir, and immediately remove from heat.

Serve warm.

Sautéed Seafood Cantonese

We adore Chinese food and we love knowing that we can have this dish any time we want it.

4	tablespoons olive oil	1	teaspoon dried basil
½	pound sea scallops, diced	½	teaspoon dried tarragon
¼	pound shrimp, diced	½	teaspoon dried thyme
¼	pound crabmeat, diced	1½	tablespoons fresh lemon juice
1	teaspoon minced garlic		
¼	teaspoon hot pepper flakes		

Place 3 tablespoons of olive oil in a large skillet over high heat. Add seafood.

Reduce heat to medium and cook about 5 minutes, stirring occasionally and being careful not to overcook seafood.

Heat the remaining 1 tablespoon of oil in a sauté pan over medium-high heat. Sauté the garlic and pepper flakes, moving the pan continuously.

Immediately add the seafood and sauté, moving continuously, until almost cooked.

Sprinkle the basil, tarragon, and thyme over the seafood. Drizzle with the lemon juice and serve immediately.

"Down Under" Grilled Fish

Some of the ships that take you out to the Great Barrier Reef anchor on luxurious pontoons on which they offer the most amazing buffets. This variation on one of their traditional meals works well because of the unusual blend of lime, mustard, and ginger flavors.

¼ cup lime juice

3 tablespoons olive oil

1 teaspoon Dijon mustard

2 teaspoons grated fresh gingerroot

¼ teaspoon cayenne pepper

black pepper

4 fish steaks

In a bowl, combine the lime juice, 1 tablespoon olive oil, mustard, ginger, cayenne pepper, and enough ground black pepper to suit your taste.

Add fish steaks and marinate for 45 to 60 minutes, turning steaks carefully 2 or 3 times.

Preheat broiler.

Place the fish steaks onto a broiler pan brushed with remaining 2 tablespoons olive oil and broil until center of the fish steaks is opaque and flakes with a fork, usually 5 minutes per side.

176 ❖ The Carbohydrate Addict's Cookbook

Dijon Mustard Fish

We like to use mustard as a cooking ingredient, not just as a
condiment. When you heat it up, the flavor permeates the fish
and gives it a special kick.

1 clove garlic, minced	fresh basil, chopped fine
¼ cup Dijon mustard	
½ cup dry white wine (or water)	4 medium fish fillets

In a small bowl, combine garlic, mustard, wine (or water), and basil.

Dip fillets into the mixture, completely coating the fish.

Heat medium nonstick skillet over high heat, until it is very hot.

Put the fish onto pan surface and brown on one side, about 2 minutes.

Turn the fish and cook for another few minutes. Test the fish with a fork to make certain that it flakes.

Fish 'n Vegetables on the Road

When we're traveling by car, we prepare this recipe the night before, store it in a plastic container, and enjoy this spicy one-dish vegetable and protein mixture cold.

1 pound flounder fillets	1 tablespoon lemon juice
2 tablespoons olive oil	1/2 teaspoon salt
1 tablespoon minced garlic	1/2 teaspoon dried basil
3 cups chopped cauliflower florets	1/4 teaspoon freshly ground black pepper
1 cup sliced green bell peppers	dash hot pepper sauce
2 tablespoons dry sherry	1/4 cup grated Parmesan cheese

Preheat oven to 350°F.

Place fillets in a layer in a 9-inch baking dish brushed with 1 tablespoon olive oil.

In a small saucepan over medium heat, sauté garlic, cauliflower, and green pepper in remaining 1 tablespoon olive oil until crisp-tender, and then spoon over fillets.

Combine sherry, lemon juice, salt, basil, pepper, and pepper sauce and pour mixture over fillets.

Bake, uncovered, for 25 to 30 minutes.

Remove vegetables and fish to heated platter.

Pour pan juices over fish and vegetables and sprinkle with Parmesan cheese.

SALADS

When we were young, we both considered the wilted green lettuce leaf that made its way into our sandwich as proof positive that we were eating our greens. Now we know differently. We have discovered that the best salads include unique and surprising combinations of ingredients that can tempt, please, and satisfy.

If you find that you are tired of "the same old salad," you may need some help and encouragement. Here are some of our favorite recipes.

Zippy Spinach and Green Bean Salad

This was one of Richard's standards before we met. We both brought our love of cooking and our recipes to the marriage and, in the end, it has all worked out just beautifully.

4 cups spinach leaves, washed and patted dry	3 tablespoons olive oil
6 strips bacon*	½ teaspoon teriyaki sauce*
1½ cups mushrooms, thinly sliced	salt to taste
½ cup green beans, cut into 1-inch pieces	2 hard-boiled eggs, chopped
	dash paprika

Refrigerate spinach to chill.

Cook bacon until crisp; drain on paper towels, then crumble.

Tear spinach into coarse pieces and toss with bacon, mushrooms, and green beans.

Combine olive oil, teriyaki sauce, and salt and sprinkle over the salad.

Top with chopped egg and serve with a sprinkle of paprika.

*Most recent Carbohydrate Addict's books may contain alternative guidelines for this ingredient. Consult your book's food lists for guidance. Use acceptable alternative as appropriate.

Creamy Cucumber Salad

SERVES 6

This salad is a variation on the Indian side dish, raita. We replaced the traditional high-carb yogurt that is usually an ingredient in this dish with sour cream instead. We love to include this salad when we're having a low-carb curry dish or any other spicy meal.

3 cucumbers	1 tablespoon scallions, finely chopped
1 teaspoon salt	
2 cups white vinegar	1 tablespoon fresh ginger-root, finely chopped
1 cup sour cream	
1 teaspoon sesame oil	

Peel cucumbers and slice thinly.

Mix remaining ingredients and pour over cucumbers. Stir carefully.

Chill overnight before serving.

Curried Chicken and Beef Salad

SERVES 4

When two people are doing the cooking, things can take an unexpected turn. This recipe came to be when the two of us set out to make two different salads. Eventually, we realized what we were doing and decided to join forces. The mixture turned out to be better than either of the individual parts (but that's true for the two of us, as well).

½ cup mayonnaise

1 teaspoon fresh lemon juice

2 tablespoons curry powder

1 cup cooked chicken, cut into bite-size pieces

1 cup cooked beef, cut into bite-size pieces

¼ cup diced celery

½ cup diced green beans

¼ cup diced cauliflower

2 hard-boiled eggs, halved and chilled

Blend mayonnaise, lemon juice, and curry powder.
Mix in remaining ingredients except eggs.
Chill at least 1 hour before serving to blend flavors.
Serve with hard-boiled egg halves on bed of lettuce.

Green Salad and Chicken Livers

No one could have convinced us that cream and liver go together until we tasted this!

⅓ cup heavy cream	½ pound chicken livers
1 teaspoon Dijon mustard	3 cups romaine lettuce, torn
¼ teaspoon salt	1 hard-boiled egg, chopped
pinch white pepper	

In a medium frying pan combine cream, mustard, salt, and pepper.

Bring to a boil over medium-high heat, stirring until cream is reduced by about a third.

Add livers, stirring gently to coat with cream. Reduce heat to medium and cook, turning occasionally, until the liquid forms a glaze that clings to the livers and the livers are cooked through.

Remove from heat and let stand until livers are warm, not hot.

In a large bowl, mix lightly with the romaine and your favorite salad dressing,* sprinkle with chopped eggs and serve.

*As per our low-carbohydrate program guidelines.

Marinated Cauliflower Salad

This recipe was born of necessity. We had the opportunity to spend time in a rainforest in Australia but had no time to prepare food. The food table they set up was full of carbs. We had two cans of tuna in our camera case for just such emergencies (don't even ask!) but we needed a vegetable to make our lunch complete. Here's the memorable dish that we discovered when we added all the condiments available to the only low-carb food on the table. We've been enjoying it ever since.

1 pound cauliflower florets, cut into bite-size pieces	$^1/_8$ teaspoon white pepper
water	$^1/_2$ cup chopped celery
$^1/_4$ cup white vinegar	3 tablespoons olive oil
1 teaspoon Dijon mustard	chopped parsley for garnish
$^1/_4$ teaspoon salt	

Add cauliflower to 2 inches of water in a small pan. Heat over a high heat and boil for 5 to 7 minutes.

Place in a colander and rinse with cold water to stop cooking. Drain well and place in a shallow bowl.

In a small bowl, combine vinegar, mustard, salt, pepper, and celery.

Using a whisk or fork, gradually beat in oil until well combined.

Pour dressing over cauliflower, cover, and refrigerate 6 to 8 hours or overnight.

Serve cold with favorite meat, chicken, or fish dish, garnished with parsley.

Steak Salad Western Style

We call this dish our bachelor's delight because when our friend
Al separated from his wife, this was his idea of gourmet cooking!

4 4- to 6-ounce pieces
   sirloin steak, trimmed

2 green bell peppers, cut in
   $1/4$-inch strips

1 small onion, chopped

$1/2$ pound green beans, ends
   trimmed and blanched

Preheat broiler.

Arrange steaks on a foil-lined baking pan. Broil 6 minutes per side.

When cooked through, remove the steaks and place in a suitable container, cover, and refrigerate.

When the meat is cold and ready to serve, cut it into $1/4$-inch strips.

In large mixing bowl, place steak strips, green pepper, onion, and green beans.

Toss with mayonnaise or your favorite salad dressing* and serve.

---

*As per our low-carbohydrate program guidelines.

New Spinach Salad with Vinaigrette

SERVES 4

Richard loves to experiment and we never know what he's going to put together. The warm broth in this salad wilts the spinach just perfectly, and adds a savory, comfy flavor.

2 tablespoons olive oil	black pepper to taste
4 tablespoons white vinegar	1 teaspoon oregano
4 tablespoons warm chicken stock, homemade only (page 26), or water	1 teaspoon chopped chives
	8 cups spinach leaves, washed, dried, and torn

In a small bowl, combine olive oil, vinegar, and chicken stock.

Add herbs immediately before serving (to enhance differences in flavors).

Toss with spinach and serve.

Betty's Garden Surprise

In her organic garden, our friend Betty grows the most wonderful vegetables on Block Island. For all the years that we lived there, Sundays at Betty's meant a special salad, fresh from the garden—a warm and wonderful meal, followed by a hot game of cards!

²/₃ cup sour cream	2 cups alfalfa sprouts
¹/₃ cup mayonnaise	¹/₂ medium cucumber, thinly sliced
2 teaspoons Dijon mustard	
³/₄ pound spinach, washed and dried, stems removed	¹/₂ cup diced celery
	¹/₂ cup diced cauliflower
6 ounces mushrooms, sliced	¹/₂ cup diced green bell pepper

In a small bowl, mix sour cream, mayonnaise, and mustard until smooth and well combined. Cover and refrigerate for 1 hour or longer to blend flavors.

In a salad bowl, combine spinach, mushrooms, sprouts, cucumber, celery, and cauliflower. Set aside.

Before serving, add sour cream mixture to the vegetables and toss lightly.

Garnish with diced green peppers.

Swiss Spinach Salad

We were almost out of money but unwilling to cut our New Zealand adventure short, so we bought the little food that we could afford, supplemented it with condiments from the free fixings bar, and discovered that, sometimes, the best things in life are nearly free.

³/₄ pound spinach leaves, washed and dried, stems removed	¹/₄ teaspoon salt
	¹/₄ teaspoon dried tarragon
	dash black pepper
1 egg yolk*	¹/₂ cup olive oil
2 tablespoons white vinegar	6 ounces mushrooms, thinly sliced
1 teaspoon Dijon mustard	¹/₂ cup diced Swiss cheese
¹/₂ teaspoon minced garlic	2 hard-boiled eggs, grated

Tear spinach leaves into bite-size pieces and place in a large bowl. Set aside.

In a small bowl, beat egg yolk with vinegar, mustard, garlic, salt, tarragon, and pepper. Gradually blend in the olive oil. Add ²/₃ of the mixture to the bowl with the spinach and mix lightly.

Arrange spinach mixture on 4 salad plates. Garnish with mushrooms in rows on opposite sides of each portion of spinach.

Drizzle remaining olive oil mixture over mushrooms.

Scatter cheese cubes over spinach and finish by sprinkling grated eggs over cheese.

Serve at once.

*Use certified, salmonella-free eggs only.

Southern Chef's Salad

When the makers of luncheon meats started adding more sugar and glutamates, we discovered a very satisfying variation to one of our favorite salads.

3   cups cooked chicken, julienned

1   cup cooked steak, julienned

½ cup diced jalapeño cheese

1   egg yolk*

1   tablespoon white vinegar

2   teaspoons Dijon mustard
    dash cayenne pepper

⅓ cup olive oil

1   teaspoon chopped garlic

12 romaine lettuce leaves, shredded

3   hard-boiled eggs

In a large bowl, combine chicken, steak, and cheese.

In a medium bowl, beat egg yolk with vinegar, mustard, and cayenne.

Using a whisk or fork, gradually beat in olive oil until mixture is thick and creamy.

Mix in the garlic.

Combine dressing with chicken, steak, and cheese mixture.

Spoon portions onto shredded romaine on individual salad plates.

Cut eggs into wedges and garnish the salad.

*Use certified, salmonella-free eggs only.

Deborah's Confetti Salad

Richard's daughter includes this wonderful mixture as part of her healthy diet. After a good workout at the gym, she fortifies herself with this crunchy taste-pleaser. We sometimes enjoy it too—but without the workout first.

1 celery heart, thinly sliced	freshly crushed black pepper
¾ cup blue cheese, crumbled	hot sauce
¼ cup balsamic vinegar*	olive oil, optional

Mix celery and cheese, then toss with vinegar. Add pepper and hot sauce to taste. Add olive oil if desired.

*Most recent Carbohydrate Addict's books may contain alternative guidelines for this ingredient. Consult your book's food lists for guidance. Use acceptable alternative as appropriate.

Painter's Pallet Garden Salad

Shredded red cabbage adds flavor and color to this recipe and, when we're having friends over for dinner, this salad makes a very pretty centerpiece as well.

8 cups dark green leaf lettuce, torn

½ medium cucumber, sliced ⅛ inch thick

1 cup shredded red cabbage

4 cups chopped green bell pepper

2 tablespoons white vinegar

1 clove garlic, minced

¼ teaspoon dried marjoram

⅛ teaspoon salt

dash black pepper

⅓ cup olive oil

In a salad bowl, gently mix lettuce, cucumber, red cabbage, and green pepper. Chill for an hour.

While salad is chilling, place vinegar, garlic, marjoram, salt, and black pepper into a small bowl and mix thoroughly.

Gradually mix in oil until dressing is well blended and slightly thickened.

Pour olive oil mixture over chilled salad and toss gently. Serve warm.

Hearty Spinach Salad

Certain foods seem to have certain seasons. This is one of our "winter" salads; it fuels us in anticipation of harsh winds and holiday shopping.

10 ounces spinach, washed, dried, and torn

10 fresh mushrooms, sliced

4 hard-boiled eggs, chopped

6 slices bacon,* cooked and crumbled

1 cup olive oil

¼ cup sour cream

¼ cup white vinegar

½ teaspoon dry mustard

½ tablespoon salt

¼ teaspoon black pepper

In a large bowl, toss spinach, mushrooms, chopped egg, and crumbled bacon.

Whisk remaining ingredients together.

Add to bowl and toss to coat.

*Most recent Carbohydrate Addict's books may contain alternative guidelines for this ingredient. Consult your book's food lists for guidance. Use acceptable alternative as appropriate.

Spicy Cucumber Salad

Richard loves vibrant flavors; he says this salad wakes up the sleepiest taste buds!

3 cups thinly sliced peeled and seeded cucumbers

2 teaspoons salt

3 hard-boiled eggs

1 teaspoon prepared white horseradish

$^1/_2$ cup sour cream

1 tablespoon white vinegar

1 bunch spinach, rinsed well, stems removed

fresh dill sprigs for garnish

Cut cucumber slices into half-moon shapes.

Place cucumbers in a large bowl with salt and toss well. Let stand at room temperature for 25 to 30 minutes. Rinse well to remove all salt.

Meanwhile, slice eggs in half. Separate yolks and whites. Chop whites and set aside. Mash egg yolks with horse-radish, sour cream, and vinegar.

Toss together cucumbers, egg whites, and egg-yolk mixture.

Arrange spinach leaves on 4 salad plates.

Spoon cucumber salad on top. Garnish with dill sprigs.

Cobb Salad

SERVES 6 TO 8

Guests of the Oprah Winfrey Show stay at the Omni Hotel in Chicago. Each time we appeared on her show, we delighted in the hotel restaurant's superb Cobb Salad. Here's our low-carb version that we enjoy at home.

6 cups green leaf lettuce, torn

3 cups chicory greens, torn

2 cucumbers, diced

4 celery stalks, chopped

2 cups mushrooms, sliced

½ pound bacon,* fried crisp and crumbled

2 cups cooked chicken, diced

1 cup crumbed blue cheese

½ pound Swiss cheese, diced

4 hard-boiled eggs, chopped

In a large bowl combine lettuce and chicory.

Top greens with lines of cucumber, celery, mushrooms, bacon, chicken, blue cheese, Swiss cheese, and eggs.

Serve with oil and vinegar.

*Most recent Carbohydrate Addict's books may contain alternative guidelines for this ingredient. Consult your book's food lists for guidance. Use acceptable alternative as appropriate.

Tangy Cauliflower Salad

When people need to add new life to their low-carb meals, we give them this recipe and explain that it fills our need for something with "bite."

1 head cauliflower, washed	1 tablespoon Dijon mustard
salt to taste	
ground black pepper to taste	$^1/_2$ cup olive oil
	1 small green chile pepper
$^1/_3$ cup white vinegar	$^1/_4$ teaspoon red pepper flakes
$1^1/_2$ tablespoons teriyaki sauce*	

Cut cauliflower head into small florets. Cook florets in boiling, salted water until tender, about 4 minutes. Drain. Season with salt and pepper.

In a small bowl, stir together the vinegar, teriyaki sauce, and mustard. Slowly whisk in the olive oil.

Seed and mince chile pepper and add to the dressing.

Serve immediately or store cauliflower and dressing separately in the refrigerator. If stored overnight, prior to serving bring dressing and cauliflower to room temperature, toss dressing and cauliflower together, sprinkle with red pepper flakes, and serve.

*Most recent Carbohydrate Addict's books may contain alternative guidelines for this ingredient. Consult your book's food lists for guidance. Use acceptable alternative as appropriate.

Popeye's Triumph

SERVES 4 TO 6

Though this salad takes a little bit of planning, the blend of flavors makes it well worth it. We always prepare enough of the dressing to last for several days and use it to baste meats, fish, and chicken as well.

1 teaspoon prepared mustard

2 tablespoons white vinegar

2 teaspoons lemon juice

½ cup olive oil

½ cup grated Parmesan cheese

salt to taste

ground black pepper to taste

1 large bunch spinach, washed and patted dry

1 cup chopped green bell pepper

⅓ cup chopped celery

In a small bowl blend together mustard, vinegar, and lemon juice. Add olive oil gradually, whisking constantly.

Whisk in ¼ cup of the Parmesan cheese. Season with salt and pepper. Cover and set aside for at least 1 hour or up to 1 day.

Tear spinach into large bowl. Add green pepper, celery, and dressing. Toss to coat well.

Add remaining ¼ cup Parmesan, toss to blend, and serve.

Celery Salad with Horseradish

It's easy to assume that all low-carb salads must include lettuce. Some of our favorites, like this one, contain no lettuce at all but are still low-carb and delicious.

8	ounces sour cream	2	tablespoons water
1	teaspoon prepared white horseradish	6	celery stalks, cut into $1/2$-inch slices
1	clove garlic, minced		

In a medium bowl, combine sour cream, horseradish, and garlic.

Thin mixture with water and gently stir in celery slices. Refrigerate overnight. Serve cold.

Triton's Gift

We love this salad because it makes the sweet taste of the lobster go farther.

9 cups mixed greens, washed and torn	black pepper to taste
6 tablespoons olive oil	2 tablespoons lemon juice
2 cloves garlic, crushed	1 tablespoon dried basil
1½ pounds cooked lobster meat, shredded	1 tablespoon chopped scallions
salt to taste	1 tablespoon dried tarragon
	½ tablespoon teriyaki sauce*

Place greens in large serving bowl or individual salad bowls and set aside.

In a skillet over medium heat, warm the olive oil and garlic.

Add the lobster meat and stir continually while warming for 2 minutes.

Remove from the heat, add salt, pepper, lemon juice, basil, scallions, tarragon, and teriyaki sauce and mix thoroughly.

Serve warm on greens or refrigerate and serve cold.

*Most recent Carbohydrate Addict's books may contain alternative guidelines for this ingredient. Consult your book's food lists for guidance. Use acceptable alternative as appropriate.

Taco Spinach Salad

If you've ever wanted a taco for your low-carb meal, you'll understand why we count on this salad when we're in the mood for a low-carb Mexican dish.

8 cups spinach, washed, patted dry, and torn

2 green bell peppers, chopped

2 cucumbers, sliced thin

2 tablespoons olive oil

2 cloves garlic

1 pound ground beef

   dash hot sauce

1 pound Cheddar cheese, chopped

In a large bowl, combine the spinach, peppers, and cucumbers. Toss and set aside.

In small frying pan, heat olive oil and garlic. Add ground beef and sauté until brown and cooked entirely. Add dash of hot sauce.

Remove from heat, top with cheese and cover until cheese softens and begins to melt, about 2 minutes.

Quickly add to salad mixture and serve immediately with oil and vinegar.

Green and White Delight

Richard's brother was coming to visit but somehow he had given us the wrong dates and there he was at the door! We threw this salad together from the ingredients we had in the refrigerator. We later found that the flavors are even richer if you let them blend overnight.

1 cup sour cream

1 tablespoon prepared white horseradish

½ teaspoon minced garlic

2 tablespoons water

2 cups green beans, trimmed

1 cup thinly sliced cucumbers

1 cup slivered green bell peppers

In a medium bowl, combine sour cream, horseradish, and garlic.

Thin mixture with water and gently stir in all other ingredients.

Refrigerate overnight.

Serve cold.

Abalone Salad Delight

Certain types of seafood tend to get ignored a bit. We love this unusual treat. You may have to special-order the abalone, but it's well worth it. If you want, you can use conch instead.

2 cucumbers, cut into thin slices
1 can abalone, cut into strips
1 6½-ounce can minced clams

4 tablespoons olive oil
1 clove garlic, minced
salt to taste
black pepper to taste
juice from ½ lemon

To assemble the salad, place two or three overlapping rows of cucumber slices down the center of an oval or oblong serving platter.

Add abalone strips in a crisscross pattern over the cucumber slices.

Drain the minced clams, reserving liquid for the dressing. Scatter the minced clams over platter. Set aside.

In a jar or appropriate container, combine olive oil, garlic, salt, pepper, lemon juice, and reserved clam juice. Cover and shake well.

Refrigerate salad and dressing separately until ready to serve.

Immediately prior to serving, drizzle dressing over platter.

Christmas Cabbage Salad

The red and green of the vegetables in this salad may be the reason why this dish got its name. Or perhaps it is named for some tradition that has been lost over the years. Whatever the reason, this was always served on the holiday table of Richard's best childhood friend.

1 pound green cabbage, shredded	$^1/_3$ cup olive oil
$^1/_2$ pound red cabbage, shredded	3 tablespoons white vinegar salt to taste black pepper to taste
2 tablespoons chopped fresh parsley	1 green bell pepper, sliced into rings

In a large salad bowl, combine green and red cabbages, and parsley. Set aside.

In a small bowl whisk together oil, vinegar, salt, and black pepper.

Pour dressing over cabbage and toss until thoroughly coated.

Arrange green pepper slices on top. Cover and chill before serving.

New Orleans Surprise

Our first trip together was to a conference in New Orleans, where Richard was presenting a research paper. We didn't have much money but we splurged on an expensive New Orleans restaurant that featured a variation of this dish.

1 tablespoon olive oil	2 teaspoons Dijon mustard
1 clove garlic, minced	¹/₂ teaspoon salt
¹/₂ pound shrimp, shells removed, washed and drained	¹/₈ tablespoon white pepper
	4 cups fresh spinach, washed, patted dry, and torn
¹/₃ cup heavy cream	

In a medium skillet, add oil and sauté garlic and shrimp. Cook shrimp until thoroughly done (about 8 minutes).

Add cream, mustard, salt, and pepper to skillet. Remove shrimp and set aside. Bring to a boil over medium-high heat, stirring until cream is reduced by about a third.

Remove from heat and let stand until shrimp are barely warm.

Toss shrimp and dressing with torn spinach and serve immediately.

California Greek Salad

A small restaurant in Los Angeles serves this salad at their patio tables that overlook the freeway. It isn't the most scenic place in the world but they do know how to make a wonderful salad.

2 green bell peppers, cut into 1-inch pieces

2 cucumbers, cut into 1-inch cubes

4 cauliflower florets, chopped

2 celery stalks, cut into 1-inch pieces

1/2 pound feta cheese, crumbled into bite-size pieces

1/2 teaspoon salt

black pepper to taste

3 tablespoons white vinegar

1/4 cup olive oil

In a 2-quart bowl, mix peppers, cucumber, cauliflower, celery, and feta cheese.

Season with salt, black pepper, vinegar, and olive oil.
Serve on large lettuce leaves or spinach leaves.

Mock Caesar Salad

*We love this variation on a favorite classic, made, this time,
without Caesar Salad's traditional raw eggs.*

3 tablespoons white vinegar

1 teaspoon grated lemon
zest

2 tablespoons fresh lemon
juice

1 clove garlic, peeled and
pressed

1 teaspoon Dijon mustard

2 ounces anchovy fillets,
finely chopped

2 hard-boiled eggs, finely
chopped

2 tablespoons grated
Parmesan cheese

coarsely ground black
pepper to taste

½ cup olive oil

1 head romaine lettuce, torn
into pieces

In a large bowl, combine the vinegar, lemon zest and
juice, garlic, mustard, anchovies, eggs, cheese, and pepper.
Mix well.

Slowly blend in the olive oil, stirring continually until
the mixture is emulsified.

Place the torn lettuce into a serving bowl. Toss well
with the dressing and serve immediately.

Dilly Cucumber Salad

Rachael's grandfather used to eat this salad with his sandwiches every day. He was a carpenter and Rachael's hero. After all, when you're five years old, what could be more impressive than someone who actually builds other people's houses?

2 cucumbers, peeled and sliced	coarsely ground black pepper to taste
¼ cup white vinegar	2 tablespoons fresh dill, chopped
salt to taste	

Place the cucumber slices in a large bowl.

Add the vinegar, salt, pepper, and dill and mix well.

Serve immediately or store covered in the refrigerator for 2 to 4 hours before serving.

Shrimp and Mushroom Salad

If anyone had ever told us that we would enjoy a dish that combined shrimp and sour cream, we wouldn't have believed it. But our friend Lynn made us try her invention and it was love at first bite.

4 cups fresh mushrooms	$^1/_3$ cup mayonnaise
1 pound shrimp, cooked, cleaned, and cooled	1 tablespoon lemon juice
$^3/_4$ cup chopped celery	$^3/_4$ teaspoon curry powder
$^1/_2$ cup sour cream	$^1/_4$ teaspoon pepper
	$^1/_8$ teaspoon salt

In a large bowl, combine mushrooms, shrimp, and celery.

In a medium bowl, combine sour cream, mayonnaise, lemon juice, curry powder, pepper, and salt, stirring well.

Add the sour cream mixture to the mushroom, shrimp, and celery mixture and toss to coat.

Refrigerate for 1 hour and serve.

King Crab Salad

Rachael's cousin ate virtually nothing but this salad when she was pregnant. Rachael thought the crab and Parmesan cheese combination sounded less than appetizing until she tried it herself and loved it. Her cousin hasn't eaten it since the baby was born.

6 cups romaine lettuce or spinach, washed, patted dry, and torn

2 tablespoons white vinegar

1/2 teaspoon lemon juice

2 tablespoons Dijon mustard

1 clove garlic, minced

1/4 teaspoon salt

dash black pepper

1/3 cup olive oil

1 tablespoon chopped parsley

1 16-ounce can king crab, drained

1/4 cup grated Parmesan cheese

Place greens in a large salad bowl and set aside.

In a medium bowl, combine vinegar, lemon juice, mustard, garlic, salt, and pepper.

Gradually blend in olive oil, mixing until well combined and slightly thickened. Stir in parsley.

Sprinkle evenly with crab and Parmesan cheese and serve on salad greens. Toss before eating.

Green Mayonnaise Salad

Odd color, great taste!

1 cup mayonnaise
¼ cup minced celery
8 fresh parsley sprigs
1 tablespoon capers
1 tablespoon oregano
1 tablespoon tarragon

ground black pepper to taste
2 cups diced celery
2 cups diced green beans
2 cups diced cauliflower
2 cups diced cucumber

In a blender, mix mayonnaise, celery, parsley, capers, oregano, and tarragon until smooth. Season with pepper and put aside.

In a large bowl, combine celery, green beans, cauliflower, and cucumber.

Add the mayonnaise mixture and toss well.

Serve chilled.

VEGETABLES

Ahhh, vegetables! The prior bane of our existence has now become of the joy of our meals. We make certain to never overcook them—always serve them raw or lightly cooked and still crisp.

We consider vegetables fair game for a good stir-fry, to be topped with cheese, spread with dips, or combined with sauce. You'll never find a naked, limp, steamed veggie at our table.

Creamy Veggie Supreme

On winter weekend afternoons, we love this warm and rich recipe served up with a beef or chicken dish.

4 large celery stalks, chopped	¼ cup sour cream
½ head cauliflower, washed and chopped	¼ cup chopped fresh parsley
	½ teaspoon dry mustard
⅓ pound crisply cooked bacon,* crumbled	½ teaspoon salt
	¼ teaspoon coarsely ground black pepper
½ cup heavy cream	

Place the celery and cauliflower into a large bowl and set aside.

In a medium bowl, combine bacon, cream, sour cream, parsley, mustard, salt, and pepper. Mix until smooth.

Pour mixture over the celery and cauliflower and toss until all of the vegetables are coated.

Serve immediately.

---

*Most recent Carbohydrate Addict's books may contain alternative guidelines for this ingredient. Consult your book's food lists for guidance. Use acceptable alternative as appropriate.

James's Roasted Capsicums

SERVES 4

Our adaptation of a luscious low-carb recipe that a young Australian white-water rafting river guide served up with snaggers—hot lamb sausages.

4   large green bell peppers,   2   teaspoons fresh lemon
    halved lengthwise   juice

2   tablespoons extra virgin
    olive oil

Preheat broiler.

Line a baking sheet with aluminum foil. Remove pepper stems and seeds.

Using the palm of your hand, flatten the pepper halves. Lay the peppers, skin side up, in a single layer on the baking sheet. Place under the broiler 3 to 4 inches from the heat source and broil 12 to 15 minutes or until the skins are charred.

Remove the peppers to a paper or plastic bag, close tightly, and let the peppers steam for about 15 minutes. Remove the peppers from the bag and remove and discard the skins.

Place the peppers in a dish and sprinkle with the olive oil and lemon juice. Gently coat the peppers on both sides.

Cover and refrigerate until ready to use. When ready to serve, allow the peppers to come to room temperature.

Beefy Asparagus and Cabbage

*We enjoy this quick variation. A simple vacation from plain
steamed veggies, it's great cold, too.*

12 asparagus spears, woody stems removed	¼ head green cabbage, shredded
1 tablespoon olive oil	lemon juice to taste
8 ounces ground beef	coarse salt to taste
2 cloves garlic, chopped	

Peel the outer layer from the bottom half of each asparagus spear. Put spears aside.

Heat the olive oil in a large skillet over medium-high
heat. Add ground beef and garlic and brown.

Add cabbage and sauté until cabbage becomes limp.

Add asparagus and sauté until asparagus is bright
green, 2 to 3 minutes.

Serve sprinkled with lemon juice and salt to taste.

Broccoli Surprise

We find that the sour cream sauce in this recipe sparks up any low-carb meal. Great with crab or shrimp. Use any low-carb vegetable instead of broccoli, if you like.

4   cups broccoli florets*

1   tablespoon lemon juice

$\frac{1}{8}$ teaspoon salt

    pinch ground black
    pepper

$\frac{1}{4}$ teaspoon dried basil

$\frac{1}{4}$ teaspoon dried
    tarragon

$\frac{1}{2}$ cup sour cream

Steam broccoli over medium-high heat for 5 to 7 minutes; drain and cool slightly.

In a bowl, combine remaining ingredients.

Toss with broccoli and serve immediately.

*Most recent Carbohydrate Addict's books may contain alternative guidelines for this ingredient. Consult your book's food lists for guidance. Use acceptable alternative as appropriate.

Spicy Creamed Spinach

We add chunks of leftover cooked chicken or steak for a satisfying one-dish meal.

1 pound chopped fresh spinach, washed and stemmed or 1 package frozen chopped spinach, defrosted and drained

pinch salt

pinch ground black pepper

1/2 cup grated jalapeño cheese or cheese of choice

1/4 cup sour cream

Steam spinach for 2 minutes and cool slightly.

In bowl, combine remaining ingredients, add spinach, and toss well.

Serve warm or cold.

Traditional Cabbage Slaw

*We enjoy this "legal" low-carb variation with burgers hot from
the grill and a dill pickle.*

2 cups shredded cabbage	1 tablespoon olive oil
1/2 green bell pepper, cut into strips	1 tablespoon white vinegar
1/3 cup chopped chives	1/4 teaspoon salt
1/4 cup thinly sliced fresh basil leaves	1/8 teaspoon pepper

In a large bowl, combine all of the ingredients and mix
thoroughly.

Refrigerate for 2 hours and serve.

Cheddar Cabbage

We invented this dish on a rainy November afternoon. It warmed and satisfied us and we hope it does the same for you.

2 tablespoons olive oil

4 cups coarsely chopped cabbage

1 cup diced celery

½ cup chopped chives

1 cup milk or cream

¼ cup Cheddar cheese

¼ teaspoon salt

2 eggs, lightly beaten

1 egg white

2 tablespoons minced fresh parsley

1 tablespoon grated Parmesan cheese

Preheat oven to 375°F.

Heat 1 tablespoon olive oil in a small skillet over medium heat. Add cabbage, celery, and chives and sauté 7 to 8 minutes, or until tender.

Coat a 10 by 6-inch baking dish with remaining 1 tablespoon olive oil and add cabbage mixture.

In a medium bowl, combine milk, Cheddar cheese, salt, eggs, and egg white, stirring well. Pour over cabbage mixture.

Combine parsley and Parmesan cheese and sprinkle over cabbage mixture.

Bake for 40 to 45 minutes. Let stand 5 minutes before serving.

Seasoned Mushrooms

As a special treat, we add shrimp to this tangy side dish or serve it with a crabmeat salad.

1 pound mushrooms	1 teaspoon grated lemon zest
$\frac{1}{2}$ cup olive oil	
2 cloves garlic, minced	1 bay leaf
1 teaspoon salt	$1\frac{1}{2}$ tablespoons lemon juice
$\frac{1}{8}$ teaspoon white pepper	$\frac{1}{4}$ cup white vinegar
$\frac{1}{2}$ teaspoon dried thyme	chopped parsley

Rinse mushrooms and pat dry.

Heat olive oil in a frying pan over medium heat and cook mushrooms for 3 minutes, stirring constantly.

Add garlic, salt, pepper, thyme, lemon zest, bay leaf, lemon juice, and vinegar.

Stir constantly for 3 minutes, then remove from heat. Transfer contents to a glass bowl and refrigerate overnight.

Top with parsley and serve cold.

Chili Spinach

This delicious dish has kept us warm through many a cold winter's day!

2 or 3 dashes chili powder
1 tablespoon olive oil
1 clove garlic, minced
1 pound fresh spinach, washed and stemmed, or 1 package frozen spinach, defrosted and drained

¹/₄ teaspoon salt
¹/₄ teaspoon ground black pepper

In a small dish, combine chili powder and olive oil. Mix well.

Heat the chili oil mixture in a large Dutch oven or wok over medium-high heat.

Add garlic and sauté 1 minute.

Carefully add spinach, salt, and pepper and toss.

Cook 5 to 6 minutes (less if using frozen spinach), stirring well 2 or 3 times during the cooking.

Serve.

Mushroom and Celery Succotash

Richard invented this one afternoon to spice up a tuna salad lunch. We've been enjoying it ever since.

2	tablespoons olive oil	1	tablespoons teriyaki sauce*
4	celery stalks, cut into ¼-inch slices	1	pound mushroom caps, sliced
3	scallions, diced		salt to taste
1	tablespoon chopped fresh parsley		ground black pepper to taste

In a frying pan large enough to hold all ingredients, heat the olive oil over medium heat. Add celery and sauté for 3 minutes, stirring constantly.

Add the scallions and parsley and sauté, stirring, for 1 minute. Remove mixture from pan and reserve.

Add the teriyaki sauce and raise heat to medium-high. Add mushrooms and sauté, tossing occasionally, until done, about 5 minutes.

Return celery, scallions, and parsley to the pan, and heat about 2 minutes, stirring often. Add salt and pepper, mix well, and serve immediately.

*Most recent Carbohydrate Addict's books may contain alternative guidelines for this ingredient. Consult your book's food lists for guidance. Use acceptable alternative as appropriate.

Colorful Coleslaw

We love the look of this side dish as much as the taste. We think it's a great complement for a warm pork roast or beef roast meal. When we have the time, we refrigerate this overnight to bring out the flavor even more.

1 cup mayonnaise	3 cups shredded green cabbage
3 teaspoons white vinegar	
1/4 teaspoon celery seeds	2 cups shredded red cabbage
1/4 teaspoon salt	
1/8 teaspoon ground pepper	1/2 green bell pepper, minced

In a large bowl, combine and blend mayonnaise, vinegar, celery seeds, salt, and black pepper. Set aside.

Mix together remaining ingredients.

Pour mayonnaise mixture over cabbage mixture, toss and serve.

Sydney Harbor Spinach

We discovered this wonderful side dish while enjoying the beauty of Sydney Harbor and it always makes us just a bit nostalgic for an adventure down under.

10 cups spinach leaves, washed and torn	1 teaspoon dried dill weed
½ pound mushrooms, thinly sliced	1 tablespoon white vinegar
½ cup mayonnaise	1 teaspoon Dijon mustard
	3 tablespoons olive oil

In a medium skillet, sauté spinach and mushrooms in very little water until spinach wilts, then set aside.

Combine mayonnaise, dill weed, vinegar, and mustard in a medium bowl.

Gradually beat in oil with a whisk. Add dressing to spinach mixture and blend lightly.

Joanna's Tangy Cauliflower

An old friend sent this recipe to us from Canada and made us promise to try it before we wrote this book. She was right—it's terrific!

2 cups water	dash black pepper
2¼ teaspoons salt	3 tablespoons olive oil
1 head cauliflower, cut into bite-size pieces	½ cup chopped green bell pepper
¼ cup white vinegar	chopped parsley
1 teaspoon Dijon mustard	

Place water and 2 teaspoons of salt into a large pot over high heat. Bring salted water to a boil, add cauliflower, and cook just until crisp-tender, 5 to 7 minutes.

Drain cauliflower in a colander and rinse with cold water to stop cooking. Drain well.

In a small bowl, combine vinegar, mustard, remaining ¼ teaspoon salt, and black pepper. Gradually beat in olive oil until well combined.

Pour oil mixture over cauliflower. Cover and refrigerate 6 to 8 hours or overnight.

Just before serving, add green peppers, mixing to combine with marinade. Sprinkle with parsley and serve.

Flavorful Fennel Mushrooms

This is our adaptation of a delightful dish from our favorite Indian restaurant. The owner retired and closed it down and we still miss their one-of-a-kind meals.

½ cup olive oil

⅓ cup fresh lemon juice, strained for seeds

½ teaspoon dried thyme, crushed

1 teaspoon fennel seed

1 clove garlic, finely slivered

1 celery stalk, minced

10 black peppercorns

1 bay leaf

½ cup water

1 lemon

2 pounds mushroom caps

2 tablespoons minced fresh parsley

In a saucepan over medium heat, combine olive oil, lemon juice, thyme, fennel, garlic, celery, peppercorns, bay leaf, and water.

Bring to a boil, cover, reduce heat, and simmer for 5 minutes, until celery is just tender.

Cut lemon in half and rub mushroom caps with cut surfaces of lemon.

Add caps to simmering liquid and cook 5 minutes.

Remove bay leaf and mushrooms with slotted spoon. Discard bay leaf and arrange mushrooms on a serving dish.

Raise heat and boil liquid until it reduces and thickens.

Pour sauce over mushrooms and add parsley; cover and chill well.

Swiss Cauliflower

We depend on this recipe and enjoy it often as one of our basics.

½ cup water	½ pound imported Swiss cheese, grated
4 cups cauliflower florets	ground pepper to taste

Place the water in a large, deep skillet over high heat. Add cauliflower, cover, and heat for 5 minutes.

Turn off the heat, remove cover and pour off the water. Sprinkle the cheese over the cauliflower, cover, and let stand for 2 more minutes.

Remove the cover, add pepper to taste, and serve immediately.

Garlicky Green Beans and Mushrooms

SERVES 4 TO 6

This dish never fails to satisfy and makes us feel good all over.

½ cup water

⅛ teaspoon salt

1 pound green beans, ends trimmed

8 medium mushroom caps, sliced

¼ cup olive oil

1 clove garlic, minced

additional salt to taste

ground pepper to taste

Put the water, ⅛ teaspoon of salt, and the green beans in a deep skillet. Cover and cook over high heat until the beans become tender, about 3 minutes. Add the mushrooms and cover the skillet.

In a small saucepan over medium heat, combine the olive oil and garlic.

Place the bean and mushroom mixture in a serving dish and pour the oil-garlic mixture over the top. Add additional salt and pepper to taste and serve warm.

Crisp and Tangy Blend

We often bring this spicy, cheerful dish to barbecues or parties.

3 cups water

1/4 teaspoon salt

4 cups shredded green cabbage

2 cups diced green beans

2 small hot green chile peppers

1/8 teaspoon dried oregano

1/8 teaspoon dried basil

1 bay leaf

1 large clove garlic, quartered lengthwise

1/4 cup white vinegar

In a large bowl, combine 1 1/2 cups of water and salt. Add the cabbage and green beans and soak for 10 minutes. Drain and discard the liquid.

In a medium saucepan, combine the cabbage, beans, chile peppers, oregano, basil, bay leaf, garlic, and vinegar. Add the remaining 1 1/2 cups of water and mix well.

Place the saucepan over medium-high heat and bring the mixture to a rapid boil. Immediately remove from heat, uncover, and let cool.

Remove bay leaf.

Serve warm or chilled.

Molly's Mushrooms

When our favorite ten-year-old came back from a trip to the Middle East, she was full of wonderful stories, excitement, and a photo of her hamming it up with a camel. We were surprised to find that she brought back a special gift, just for us—the recipe for her favorite vegetarian dish. Molly has already learned that some of the best gifts take up no packing space!

1	pound mushroom caps, washed	1	celery stalk
2	cups water	1	teaspoon basil, fresh or dried
1	cup virgin olive oil	$\frac{1}{2}$	teaspoon thyme
2	cloves garlic, sliced	1	bay leaf
	juice of 1 lemon	10	black peppercorns
1	tablespoon white vinegar	$\frac{1}{2}$	teaspoon salt

In a large pot, combine all ingredients.

Bring to a boil, then turn down heat and simmer for 5 minutes, occasionally stirring mixture.

Pour into bowl and marinate overnight in refrigerator.

Place a wooden toothpick through each mushroom and serve on a bed of lettuce.

Green-Topped Cauliflower

When we're really hungry, this dish can't be beat. Great with chicken or fish.

1 cup water	3 ounces jalapeño pepper cheese, grated
1 small head cauliflower, washed and chopped	1/4 cup sour cream
1 10-ounce package frozen chopped spinach	1/4 teaspoon ground black pepper
1 tablespoon chopped chives	1/2 teaspoon minced fresh garlic
2 tablespoons olive oil	1/4 teaspoon celery salt

Place the water in a large skillet over a high heat. Add the cauliflower, cover, and heat for 4 minutes.

Drain the water and keep a lid on the skillet.

Cook spinach according to package directions; drain, retaining 1/4 cup of the cooking water.

In a medium saucepan over low heat, cook chives in olive oil until chives are limp.

Add spinach, cheese, sour cream, pepper, garlic, spinach water, and salt, stirring occasionally until cheese is melted and mixture is creamy.

Place the cauliflower in a serving dish, cover with the spinach-cheese mixture, and serve.

Asparagus-Egg-Mushroom Casserole

This casserole always makes us feel as if we aren't having a low-carb meal, yet it's perfectly "legal."

1 11-ounce can asparagus spears (or fresh equivalent, parboiled)	salt to taste
	ground black pepper to taste
1 tablespoon olive oil	1/2 cup grated Cheddar cheese
4 hard-boiled eggs, sliced	2 cloves garlic, minced
12 mushroom caps, sliced	2 large slices imported Swiss cheese
1 cup heavy cream	

Preheat oven to 350°F.

Drain asparagus.

Oil the bottom and sides of a medium casserole and arrange half the asparagus spears on bottom of casserole.

Cover with half the egg slices and half the mushroom slices.

Pour half the cream over the contents of the casserole, and add salt and pepper to taste.

Sprinkle with half Cheddar cheese and half of the minced garlic.

Repeat the process for the second layer.

Place Swiss cheese slices over all and bake for 30 minutes.

Serve warm.

Sesame Broccoli and Spinach

SERVES 4

Rachael cooked this up as a special treat for guests who never showed up. Now, we can't even remember who they were but we never forgot the recipe.

½ head broccoli,* rinsed and chopped	2 tablespoons white vinegar
2 cups water	1 tablespoon teriyaki sauce*
1½ pounds raw spinach, washed and cut into large pieces (or frozen equivalent)	1 teaspoon Dijon mustard
	2 teaspoons capers
	salt to taste
2 tablespoons sesame oil	ground black pepper to taste

Put broccoli and water in a large skillet over a high heat, cover, and let heat for 5 minutes.

Lower the heat to medium, add the spinach and continue to steam for 1 more minute. Remove the skillet from the heat, immediately add cold water to pan to immerse spinach and broccoli.

Drain and gently squeeze out as much moisture as possible. Place broccoli and spinach in a medium bowl and set aside.

In a small bowl, combine sesame oil, vinegar, teriyaki sauce, and mustard. Mix thoroughly.

Add the mixture to broccoli and spinach, toss gently and sprinkle with capers and salt and pepper to taste.

Serve warm or cold.

*Most recent Carbohydrate Addict's books may contain alternative guidelines for this ingredient. Consult your book's food lists for guidance. Use acceptable alternative as appropriate.

Super Stuffed Mushrooms

We love this satisfying side dish with a salad or all by itself.

1 pound large mushrooms	4 ounces mozzarella, diced fine
5 tablespoons olive oil	salt to taste
½ pound chicken livers	ground black pepper to taste
¼ cup dried basil	
1 tablespoon minced fresh garlic	

Remove mushroom stems; rinse, and chop stems.
Heat 3 tablespoons of olive oil in a skillet over medium-high heat. Add mushroom caps and sauté for 4 to 5 minutes. Remove and set aside.

Add the remaining 2 tablespoons olive oil and the livers to the skillet and sauté until the livers are browned. Remove the livers, chop, and set aside to cool.

Add mushroom stems, basil, livers, and garlic to the skillet and sauté for 1 minute.

Combine the mozzarella and the liver mixture, adding salt and pepper to taste.

Spoon the mixture into the mushroom caps. Placing the caps on a bed of lettuce and chill well before serving.

Mexican Green Beans

Here's our adaptation of a recipe that we discovered in a restaurant somewhere in Portland, Oregon. Our lunch was superb but we could never find our way back to the restaurant again.

1 pound green beans, trimmed, washed, and sliced into 2-inch julienne

2 tablespoons olive oil

6 scallions, chopped fine
ground black pepper to taste

1/2 teaspoon chopped fresh basil

1/4 teaspoon ground cloves

1/2 teaspoon chili powder

1 1/2 cups sour cream

Sauté green beans in olive oil in a large skillet over a high heat for 2 minutes. Remove from heat and set aside.

In a large bowl, combine scallions, pepper, basil, cloves, and 1/4 teaspoon chili powder. Blend together. Add the sour cream and mix well. Sprinkle the remaining 1/4 teaspoon chili powder on both sauce and green beans.

Serve beans in individual dishes, topped with sour cream sauce.

Diane's Mustard-Garlic Medley

The Swiss cheese in this dish adds a special nutty flavor we really enjoy. We named it after an old friend who also adds a bit of nuttiness to any occasion.

2 cloves garlic, minced

2 teaspoons Dijon mustard

2 tablespoons lemon juice

1 cup water

½ cup olive oil

2 teaspoons grated imported Swiss cheese

ground black pepper to taste

2 cups chopped cauliflower

2 cups mushroom caps, washed, trimmed, and sliced

1 cup green beans, trimmed and sliced into 2-inch julienne

In a blender, food processor, or mixing bowl, combine garlic, mustard, lemon juice, and water until well mixed.

Continue mixing while gradually adding oil. Add cheese and ground pepper to taste. Set aside.

In a large bowl, combine the cauliflower, mushrooms, and green beans.

Pour in the olive oil mixture and toss the vegetables. Refrigerate overnight, tossing once or twice.

When ready to serve, toss once more.

Kelli's Tangy Grilled Asparagus with Hollandaise Sauce

SERVES 4

This wonderful dish is as delightful as our friend Kelli, who adds creativity and love to every recipe and everything she does. Whenever we want something special, we whip this up and it seems like a holiday.

16 medium asparagus spears, trimmed

¼ cup olive oil

¼ cup white vinegar

⅔ cup butter

2 egg yolks*

1 to 2 tablespoons fresh lemon juice

Tabasco or other hot sauce to taste

Marinate asparagus spears in olive oil and vinegar for 1 hour prior to grilling.

Melt butter over low heat or in microwave. Put aside.

In food processor or mixer, blend egg yolks and add one-third of the lemon juice. Blend for 3 seconds. Add one-third of melted butter. Blend for 10 seconds. Repeat these steps until lemon juice and butter are used up.

Add Tabasco sauce to taste. Blend once more.

Serve asparagus warm or cold with warm sauce. Sauce is also a fine complement to cold chicken, meat, or seafood, or warm tofu.

*Use certified salmonella-free eggs only.

Radishy Shrimp and Cabbage Slaw

SERVES 4

Richard's aunt makes this tasty dish but keeps the recipe a secret. The hard part for us was figuring out the oregano-paprika combination. She says she's happy to see it included but wouldn't let us mention her name.

2 cups shredded cabbage	1 cup sour cream
1/2 green bell pepper, cut into strips	1 teaspoon prepared white horseradish
1/3 cup chopped chives	paprika to taste
1/4 cup thinly sliced fresh basil leaves	oregano to taste
1/4 teaspoon salt	1 pound cold steamed shrimp
1/8 teaspoon pepper	

In a large bowl, combine cabbage, bell pepper, chives, basil, salt, and pepper. Mix thoroughly and set aside.

In a medium bowl, combine sour cream, horseradish, paprika, and oregano. Add shrimp and cabbage mixture and coat completely.

Refrigerate for 2 hours.

Serve cold.

Middle Eastern Mix

We found that fennel seeds can add a new flavor and interest to many of our old favorites. It's an unusual taste and if you find it pleasing, we think that you'll be adding fennel to many of your other dishes as well.

8 medium asparagus spears, washed and trimmed	1 tablespoon minced fresh parsley
8 brussels sprouts,* washed and trimmed	1/2 cup chicken stock, home-made only (page 26), or water
1/2 pound cabbage, trimmed	black pepper to taste
2 scallions, chopped	1/2 teaspoon fennel seeds

Slice asparagus spears at an angle into pieces about 1 1/2 inches long, split brussels sprouts, and slice cabbage.

In a large skillet, combine the vegetables, scallions, and parsley. Add stock (or water) and pepper to taste.

Cover and cook over moderate heat for 5 to 6 minutes.

Just before the vegetables are done, sprinkle the fennel seeds on top.

Serve warm or cold.

*Most recent Carbohydrate Addict's books may contain alternative guidelines for this ingredient. Consult your book's food lists for guidance. Use acceptable alternative as appropriate.

Delightfully Different Green Beans

SERVES 4

Our friends in CASupport™ (our online support group) wanted
a new green bean recipe. This easy dish always pleases us and
makes us glad we've found this way of eating.*

1½ cups water
½ teaspoon salt
1 pound green (or wax)
  beans, washed and
  trimmed
2 small hot green chile
  peppers
⅛ teaspoon cumin
⅛ teaspoon oregano

⅛ teaspoon dried
  sweet basil
1 bay leaf
2 cloves garlic, quartered
  lengthwise
½ cup white vinegar
¼ cup mayonnaise
¼ cup sour cream

In a medium saucepan over a high heat, combine water,
salt, beans, chile peppers, cumin, oregano, basil, bay leaf,
garlic, and vinegar, and boil for 3 minutes exactly.
Remove from heat and let cool. Remove bay leaf.

In a small bowl, blend mayonnaise and sour cream.

Remove the beans from the liquid, place on a serving
dish, and top with the mayonnaise–sour cream mixture.

*Information on CASupport™ is available through our Web site at
www.carbohydrateaddicts.com

VEGETABLES ❖ 239

Lemon Cauliflower Surprise

Each of us swears that we invented this recipe. We're probably both wrong, but, in any case, we think you'll enjoy the wonderful blend of flavors.

1 medium cauliflower, broken into florets	2 tablespoons lemon juice
1 small onion, chopped	salt to taste
¼ cup olive oil	coarsely ground black pepper to taste
1 teaspoon sesame oil	

In a large pan, in 1 inch of water, steam the cauliflower until tender, 6 to 8 minutes.

Turn off heat, drain the florets, then return them to the hot pan.

In a separate small pan, sauté onion in olive oil and sesame oil over medium heat until onion turns dark brown and caramelizes.

Pour onion and oil on cauliflower and add lemon juice and salt and pepper to taste.

Serve warm or cold.

Three-Green Garlic Toss

Though days are busy, we especially enjoy this dish when it's prepared the night before so that the flavors blend and enhance each other. If you're tight for time, make it and enjoy it right away, but do make extra to put away for tomorrow as well.

8   medium asparagus spears, trimmed and cut into 2-inch pieces

16 green beans, trimmed and cut into 2-inch julienne

8   brussels sprouts,* washed and trimmed

½   teaspoon mild dry mustard

salt to taste

coarsely ground black pepper to taste

2   cloves garlic, finely minced

1   tablespoon white vinegar

3   tablespoons lemon juice

½   cup olive oil

In a medium bowl, combine asparagus, green beans, and brussels sprouts.

In a separate bowl or large jar, combine and mix mustard, salt, and black pepper. Add the remaining ingredients to the mixture and whisk or shake until thoroughly mixed.

Pour the mixture over the vegetables.

*Most recent Carbohydrate Addict's books may contain alternative guidelines for this ingredient. Consult your book's food lists for guidance. Use acceptable alternative as appropriate.

VEGETARIAN ALTERNATIVES

We were hesitant to put these recipes in a section by themselves. Some of the recipes that follow are old and trusted friends and we wanted to be sure that all of our readers, meat-eaters and vegetarians alike, would enjoy them. Still, we didn't want our vegetarian readers to have to sort through one more stack of recipes in pursuit of good and nourishing and fun-filled meals that meet their vegan or vegetarian needs.

So, here's to you guys. Enjoy!

Cucumber Dill Salad

When Rachael was young, there was always a variation of this side dish at picnics. It still makes her think of summertime and baseball announcers calling plays on the portable radio.

2 cucumbers, peeled and sliced

salt to taste

¼ cup white vinegar

coarsely ground black pepper to taste

2 tablespoons chopped fresh dill

Place the cucumber slices in a large bowl.
 Add the salt, vinegar, pepper, and dill and mix well.
 Store covered in the refrigerator for 2 to 4 hours.
 Serve cold.

Cheesy Broccoli Casserole

Friends and family alike often ask us to bring this dish to potluck dinners. For a nice brown crust, sprinkle some Parmesan on top and put under the broiler for a few minutes before serving.

1 cup shredded Cheddar cheese	2 tablespoons olive oil
1 cup chopped mushroom caps	¼ teaspoon salt
½ cup chopped scallions	2 cups broccoli,* washed, drained, chopped
¼ cup heavy cream	vegetable cooking spray

Preheat oven to 350°F.

In a medium saucepan over low heat, combine all ingredients except cooking spray.

Cook for 3 to 5 minutes or until cheese melts, stirring constantly.

Spoon the mixture into a 2-quart casserole coated with cooking spray.

Bake 30 minutes.

Serve warm.

*Most recent Carbohydrate Addict's books may contain alternative guidelines for this ingredient. Consult your book's food lists for guidance. Use acceptable alternative as appropriate.

Asparagus Parmesan Soup

One of the few soups we have found that can be made from low-carb foods while tasting rich and delicious. If fish is part of your diet, this makes a great complement.

12 asparagus spears

1 cup water

1 tablespoon olive oil

½ cup heavy cream

¼ cup grated Parmesan cheese

black pepper to taste

Cut woody ends from asparagus.

Bring water to boil in a sauté pan, add tips, and boil slowly for 7 to 8 minutes.

Drain and purée in a blender, adding olive oil and cream.

Empty into a bowl and stir in cheese and pepper to taste.

Manhattan Mushroom Salad

The trick to this salad is to prepare it ahead of time, if possible, so that the mushrooms can soak up the creamy dressing. We always store it covered in the refrigerator.

½ cup heavy cream
½ tablespoon lemon juice
    paprika to taste
10 medium mushroom
    caps

2 tablespoons chopped celery
1 cup watercress, stems removed

In a salad bowl combine heavy cream and lemon juice, stirring.

Season to taste with paprika.

Wash mushrooms carefully under running water and pat dry with a paper towel.

Slice mushrooms very thin into bowl and stir with dressing.

Add celery, stir, and spoon over bed of watercress.

Sautéed Green Beans

This dish is a favorite of ours. For Reward Meals, we add some toasted almonds and, voila! *green beans amandine.*

2	cups water	2	tablespoons olive oil
1	teaspoon teriyaki sauce*	4	parsley sprigs, stems removed
½	pound green beans, cleaned and halved		salt to taste
½	teaspoon lemon juice		black pepper to taste

Combine water and teriyaki sauce in a sauté pan or skillet and place over medium heat.

Add beans and cook, uncovered, 4 to 5 minutes; beans should be crisp.

Drain beans and place in a bowl.

Sprinkle lemon juice over beans and add oil, parsley, and seasoning to taste.

*Most recent Carbohydrate Addict's books may contain alternative guidelines for this ingredient. Consult your book's food lists for guidance. Use acceptable alternative as appropriate.

Basic Broccoli and Cheese

We enjoy the nutty flavor of the Swiss cheese in this dish and love to have this as a lunch or snack, along with a crisp and tasty salad.

3 large broccoli spears*	½ cup white dry wine
½ cup olive oil	black pepper to taste
1 clove garlic, diced	3 slices Swiss cheese

Wash broccoli and cut off leaves and tough stem.

Chop broccoli coarsely.

Place oil in a sauté pan or skillet; add diced garlic and cook until golden; remove garlic with a spoon.

Add broccoli, mixing with oil until pieces glisten.

Pour in wine and simmer over medium heat until tender, about 6 minutes; season to taste.

While still hot, arrange Swiss cheese over broccoli and cover for 3 minutes or until cheese melts over broccoli.

Serve warm.

*Most recent Carbohydrate Addict's books may contain alternative guidelines for this ingredient. Consult your book's food lists for guidance. Use acceptable alternative as appropriate.

Creamy Cabbage Salad

When we visit Richard's son, Jonathan, he has this salad waiting for us. Jono is a fine cook, just like his dad.

1 medium cabbage, chopped fine	3 tablespoons white vinegar
1 cup sour cream	salt to taste
2 tablespoons chopped fresh parsley	black pepper to taste
⅓ cup olive oil	1 green bell pepper, cored and cut into rings

In a large salad bowl, combine cabbage, sour cream, and parsley.

In a small bowl whisk together oil, vinegar, salt, and pepper.

Pour dressing over cabbage and toss until cabbage is thoroughly coated.

Arrange bell pepper rings on top.

Cover and chill before serving.

Deviled Eggs D'Oro

Richard made this for our first picnic. We were so much in love that we forgot to eat it. We're still that much in love (maybe more) but we've never overlooked this treat since.

4   hard-boiled eggs
3   tablespoons mayonnaise
1   teaspoon Dijon mustard

2   tablespoons finely chopped green bell pepper

Cut eggs in half lengthwise, remove yolks, and place yolks in a medium bowl. Put whites aside.

Mash egg yolks, then add mayonnaise and mustard and mix thoroughly. Fold in green pepper.

Mound egg yolk mixture in egg white cavities.

Cover and refrigerate until chilled and ready to serve.

Yanni's Greek Salad with a Twist

A few blocks from the Esplanade in Cairns, Australia, you'll find what we consider the best Greek restaurant in the world. This salad makes us think of the many meals we've enjoyed there and the friends who await our return.

2 green bell peppers, cut into 1-inch pieces

1 cucumber, cut into 1-inch cubes

2 celery stalks, cut into 1-inch pieces

¼ pound feta cheese, cut into ½-inch cubes

½ teaspoon salt

ground pepper to taste

3 tablespoons white vinegar

¼ cup oil

½ teaspoon oregano

1 tablespoon minced fresh basil

2 tablespoons lemon juice

In a large bowl, combine peppers, cucumber, celery, and feta cheese.

Season with salt, pepper, vinegar, oil, oregano, and basil.

Divide salad equally into 4 bowls, sprinkle with lemon juice and serve.

Cool Creamy Spinach

When we were kids, Horn and Hardart Automats made the best creamed spinach. The restaurants closed down years ago, but this variation lives on in our kitchen.

1 package frozen spinach,
   or 1 pound fresh

2 teaspoons salt

1 cup sour cream

1 tablespoon fresh lime
   juice

1 teaspoon cumin seed
   black pepper to taste
   paprika to taste

2 tablespoons grated
   onion

Prepare spinach according to package directions and drain. (Alternatively, wash fresh spinach and steam until fully soft, about 3 minutes, then drain).

Combine remaining ingredients in a medium bowl. Stir in spinach.

Chill at least 1 hour.

Serve cold.

Crustless Spinach Pie

About two years ago, our refrigerator was just about as empty as our stomachs. We wanted a nutritious low-carb meal that tasted like a snack and put this recipe together. We've been enjoying it ever since.

2 pounds spinach, washed, drained, and chopped or 2 packages frozen chopped spinach	1 teaspoon salt
	³/₄ cup olive oil
	1 pound feta cheese, crumbled
¹/₄ cup chopped scallions	¹/₂ cup grated Parmesan cheese
¹/₄ cup chopped fresh parsley	
¹/₄ cup chopped fresh dill	2 eggs, beaten

Preheat oven to 350°F.

Combine spinach with scallions, parsley, dill, and salt.

Let stand 10 minutes. Squeeze out moisture with your hands.

Heat ¹/₂ cup olive oil in a large skillet and stir in spinach and cheeses.

Remove from heat and cool, stirring occasionally, to room temperature. Beat eggs in with a wooden spoon.

Brush bottom and sides of a 13 by 9 by 2-inch baking dish with remaining ¹/₄ cup olive oil.

Spread spinach mixture evenly in the baking dish and bake for 1 hour.

Cut into squares and serve warm. Delicious cold as well.

Stir-Fried Vegetable Festival

Rachael was a vegetarian for several years and sometimes returns to a nonmeat menu. This is one of her favorites, hot or cold.

2 cups olive oil	1 chile pepper, seeded and chopped
½ block formed firm tofu, sliced thickly	¼ cup fresh lemon juice
3 cloves garlic, minced	2 tablespoons chopped fresh parsley
1 teaspoon grated gingerroot	1 teaspoon salt
½ head cabbage, cored and shredded	½ teaspoon ground black pepper
1 cup green beans, cut into 2-inch pieces	1 tablespoon chopped cilantro
1 cup cauliflower florets, chopped	¼ teaspoon thyme

In a wok or large skillet, heat olive oil to 375°F.

Brown tofu in olive oil and remove to paper towel to drain.

Remove olive oil and return 3 tablespoons to skillet.

Sauté garlic and gingerroot until soft.

Add the cabbage, beans, cauliflower, and chile pepper. Stir-fry until vegetables are tender-crisp.

Add lemon juice, parsley, salt, ground pepper, cilantro, thyme, and browned tofu.

Cook for an additional 5 minutes, stirring to coat vegetables and tofu with sauce.

New Zealand Vegetables and Cheese

We often took this dish along for lunch on our white-water rafting trips throughout New Zealand. It gave us something to keep paddling for!

1 cup sliced mushrooms	black pepper to taste
6 medium green bell peppers	1 cup milk
4 tablespoons olive oil	2 eggs
2 cups grated Cheddar cheese	¼ cup grated Parmesan cheese
salt to taste	parsley sprigs

Heat oven to 375° F.

Wash mushrooms and green peppers and slice them into thin slices, the length of each vegetable.

Heat 1 tablespoon olive oil in a large skillet over medium heat and sauté mushrooms until light golden.

Cook another 2 minutes and remove from heat.

In a large, deep casserole dish coated with 2 table-spoons of olive oil, form a layer of half the green peppers. Sprinkle with half of the mushrooms, then with half the Cheddar cheese. Season with salt and pepper.

Repeat the layers.

Sprinkle with the remaining 1 tablespoon of olive oil.

Mix together milk and eggs and pour over mixture.

Cover with foil and bake for 30 minutes.

Uncover and bake for 15 minutes. Sprinkle with Parmesan cheese and bake another 15 minutes.

Garnish with parsley sprigs for serving.

Cheesy Breakfast "Sausages" and Tofu Stir-Fry

SERVES 4

For some reason, most vegetarian meals contain only one meat substitute. We think that combining flavors makes a richer and more satisfying meal.

1 formed tofu block, 4 by 4 inches, cut into bite-size pieces	1 cup diced celery
	½ cup diced green beans
1 tablespoon olive oil	4 slices Cheddar cheese
4 vegetarian "sausages"*	salt to taste
	black pepper to taste

Place the tofu pieces on a plate, cover with a second plate, and place a heavy object on top of the second plate to squeeze out excess water. Let stand.

After 20 minutes, pour off the water that has been squeezed from the tofu.

Place the olive oil into a large skillet over a medium heat, add the "sausages" and sauté for 3 minutes.

Add tofu, celery, and green beans to the skillet.

Sauté the mixture for 3 to 4 minutes.

Remove from heat.

Top mixture with cheese slices and cover for 4 minutes, until cheese softens and melts.

Season with salt and pepper and serve hot.

*Low-carbohydrate textured vegetable protein "meats" should contain 4 grams or fewer of carbohydrates per average serving.

Far East Tofu

SERVES 4

We love to grow our own alfalfa sprouts. Some health food stores sell little plastic strainers for just that purpose. It's really easy to place the seeds in a little water, and in a few days you're suddenly the owner of a miniature "field" of sprouts. Make certain that your sprouts are fresh, rinsed each day as they grow, and free of mold.

1 formed tofu block, 4 by 4 inches, cut into bite-size pieces	1/2 cup bean sprouts
	1 tablespoon teriyaki sauce*
1/4 cup olive oil	1/2 teaspoon garlic powder
1 cup diced celery	1/2 teaspoon dried sweet basil
1/2 cup sliced mushrooms	1 cup alfalfa sprouts

Place the tofu pieces on a plate, cover with a second plate, and place a heavy object on top of the second plate to squeeze out excess water. Let stand.

After 20 minutes, pour off the water that has been squeezed from the tofu.

Place the olive oil in a large skillet over medium heat, add the tofu and warm for 1 minute.

In a medium bowl, combine the celery, mushrooms, bean sprouts, teriyaki, garlic, and basil; pour the mixture over the tofu.

Sauté the mixture for 3 to 4 minutes.

Decorate with alfalfa sprouts and serve warm or prepare in advance and serve cold for breakfast or lunch.

*Most recent Carbohydrate Addict's books may contain alternative guidelines for this ingredient. Consult your book's food lists for guidance. Use acceptable alternative as appropriate.

Cauliflower and Broccoli with Spicy Dressing

SERVES 8

Richard's brother, Rudy, used to live on this recipe when he was a bachelor. It kept him fit and happy enough to find the woman of his dreams.

1 head cauliflower, cut into 1-inch pieces	³/₄ cup olive oil
1 bunch broccoli,* cut into 1-inch pieces	1 tablespoon lemon juice
	1 tablespoon white vinegar
4 cloves garlic	1 teaspoon salt
1 egg†	¹/₈ teaspoon white pepper
1 tablespoon Dijon mustard	capers (optional)

Place broccoli and cauliflower pieces in a steamer basket over boiling water (or in 1 inch of water in a covered pan).

Steam for 6 to 8 minutes, until a knife inserted will easily pierce vegetable.

Remove vegetables and cool.

To prepare the accompanying creamy garlic dressing, place garlic in a food processor and purée.

Add egg and mustard and then pour in a thin stream of olive oil until mixture is slightly thickened.

Season with lemon juice, vinegar, salt, and pepper.

Toss vegetables with dressing and serve. Capers may be sprinkled on top to add a little zest.

*Most recent Carbohydrate Addict's books may contain alternative guidelines for this ingredient. Consult your book's food lists for guidance. Use acceptable alternative as appropriate.
† Use certified salmonella-free eggs only.

Aromatic Tofu

This recipe is a reliable old friend we are happy to share with you.

¼ cup water	1 clove garlic, minced
2 celery stalks with leaves, rinsed	1 teaspoon ground ginger
	¼ cup teriyaki sauce*
1 cup cauliflower florets, chopped	½ tablespoon lemon juice
⅓ cup olive oil	2 formed tofu blocks, 4 by 4 inches each

In a blender, combine water and celery and make a purée.

In a large bowl, combine the celery purée, cauliflower, olive oil, garlic, ginger, teriyaki sauce, and lemon juice to form a marinade.

Place the tofu blocks on a plate, cover with a second plate, and place a heavy object on top of the second plate.

Let stand for 10 minutes, then pour off the excess water that has been squeezed from the tofu.

Chop the tofu into bite-size pieces and place them in the marinade. Cover and refrigerate overnight.

Preheat broiler.

Drain the tofu chunks reserving marinade, place them in a shallow pan, and place under the broiler until they are nicely browned, 8 to 10 minutes.

Sprinkle the tofu with leftover marinade and serve warm.

Also delicious served cold over lettuce leaves.

---

*Most recent Carbohydrate Addict's books may contain alternative guidelines for this ingredient. Consult your book's food lists for guidance. Use acceptable alternative as appropriate.

Parsley Buttered "Steaks"

SERVES 4

This recipe is one of the easiest we know but always tastes like a gourmet treat to us. We hope you enjoy it, too.

5	tablespoons butter	4	vegetarian "steaks"*
2	teaspoons chopped fresh parsley	1	clove garlic, crushed
			lemon juice to taste

In a large mixing bowl, cream together 4 tablespoons of butter and the parsley.

Refrigerate until the mixture is solid.

Place the remaining 1 tablespoon of butter into a large frying pan over medium heat.

When the butter is melted, add the "steaks" and brown on both sides, 2 to 3 minutes per side.

Spread the garlic over both sides of the "steaks." Add a small scoop of parsley butter on top of each "steak" and serve them warm with a squirt of lemon juice to taste.

*Vegetarian meat alternatives should contain 4 grams or less of carbohydrate per average serving.

"Ham" and Cheese with Tofu

One night last year, we were craving a ham-and-cheese sandwich and this recipe was born. At our next Reward Meal we indulged and had the original object of our yearning and discovered that we enjoyed this dish a whole lot more.

1 formed tofu block, 4 by 4 inches, cut into bite-size pieces	4 slices vegetarian "ham,"* diced
1 tablespoon olive oil	8 large mushrooms, sliced
4 tablespoons chopped green bell pepper	½ teaspoon dried basil
	4 slices Cheddar cheese
	black pepper to taste

Place the tofu pieces on a plate, cover with a second plate, and place a heavy object on top of the second plate.

Let stand for 10 minutes, then pour off the excess water that has been squeezed from the tofu.

Place the olive oil in a large skillet over medium heat, add the green pepper, and sauté until soft.

Add "ham" and mushrooms and sauté for 3 to 4 minutes. Add the basil and mix well.

Add the tofu pieces to the skillet and continue to sauté for 3 to 4 more minutes.

Remove from heat, top with cheese slices, and cover for 3 to 4 minutes, until cheese is soft but not liquid.

Add the black pepper and serve warm.

*Vegetarian meat alternatives should contain 4 grams or less of carbohydrate per average serving.

262 ❖ The Carbohydrate Addict's Cookbook

Tofu with a Bite

SERVES 4

We think foods should complement your mood. We always seem to choose this dish when we have a day of slow-moving meetings and want something with a little pizzazz. It's a delicious treat served warm or cold.

2 formed tofu blocks,
  4 by 4 inches each, cut
  into bite-size pieces
1 cup white vinegar
2 tablespoons chopped
  scallions
⅛ teaspoon cinnamon
⅛ teaspoon ground allspice
⅛ teaspoon ground cloves
⅛ teaspoon ground black
  pepper
⅛ teaspoon salt
2 tablespoons olive oil
1 cup mushrooms, sliced
2 celery stalks, minced

Place the tofu blocks on a plate, cover with a second plate, and place a heavy object on top of the second plate.

Let stand for 10 minutes, then pour off the excess water that has been squeezed from the tofu.

In a large bowl, combine the vinegar, scallions, cinnamon, allspice, cloves, pepper, and salt. Add tofu. Cover and marinate overnight.

When you are ready to cook the tofu, place the olive oil, mushrooms, and celery in a deep skillet over medium-high heat and sauté until the celery starts to brown, 3 to 4 minutes.

Add the tofu and sauté for an additional 3 to 4 minutes.

Serve warm or cold.

Queenstown Spinach

A little hostel sits on the hill in Queenstown, a harbor town in New Zealand. Every night the owners make this dish for all who share their gracious table.

2 bunches fresh spinach, rinsed and drained

2 tablespoons extra virgin olive oil

2 teaspoons minced garlic

1/4 teaspoon paprika

coarse salt to taste

Pat the spinach dry and cut into 1-inch pieces.

Heat olive oil in a medium skillet over medium-high heat, add the spinach pieces, garlic, and paprika and sauté until just tender, 1 or 2 minutes.

Season with salt and serve immediately.

QUICK FIX
DISHES
and
SNACKS

On the go? All the time! Want a snack? You bet! These are a few items from our foods-in-an-instant collection that hit the spot (when that spot is more like a moving target)!

Veal with Lemony Herbs

What do you do when you have already eaten your Reward Meal and your daughter brings home an unexpected guest for dinner? The answer: quickly stir up this first-rate gourmet quality meal. (It made her happy and kept us right on our program.)

4	tablespoons olive oil		black pepper to taste
8	thin veal steaks, approximately 2 ounces each	2	tablespoons finely chopped fresh basil
	salt to taste	4	lemon wedges

Heat 2 tablespoons olive oil in a large skillet over high heat.

Rub all sides of veal lightly with remaining 2 tablespoons olive oil and season with salt and pepper.

Sear steaks quickly, about 1 minute per side.

Place veal on warmed plate.

Sprinkle with basil, garnish with lemon, and serve immediately.

Tasty Sautéed Green Peppers and Celery

SERVES 4

This dish never makes it to the table in this form. One of us will always add some leftovers or cheese as we stir things up. One afternoon, on a whim, we added chicken, cheese, mushrooms, and olives. It was quite good.

2	tablespoons olive oil	dash teriyaki sauce*
4	large celery stalks, diced	salt to taste
4	large green bell peppers, sliced in thin wedges	black pepper to taste

In a large skillet over medium heat, add olive oil and celery.

Cook over medium heat 2 to 3 minutes.

Add green peppers and stir until peppers are slightly browned, about 10 minutes. Sprinkle with teriyaki sauce and cook one more minute.

Sprinkle with salt and pepper.

*Most recent Carbohydrate Addict's books may contain alternative guidelines for this ingredient. Consult your book's food lists for guidance. Use acceptable alternative as appropriate.

Poached Lemon Salmon

Rachael depends on this recipe. It's easy to make in the evening, while we clean up the dinner dishes, so that it's cold and ready for breakfast for the next two days.

⅓ cup lemon juice	4 large salmon fillets
½ cup water	2 tablespoons minced fresh parsley
1 teaspoon minced garlic	

In a large skillet over medium-high heat, bring lemon juice and water to a boil. Add garlic.

Add salmon, lower heat to medium, and cover skillet. Cook for 5 to 8 minutes.

Salmon is done when it flakes when pressed with a fork.

Serve immediately, garnished with parsley, or chill and serve cold.

Mediterranean Olives and Asparagus

SERVES 6

Olives add a special flavor that we both enjoy. We love this dish with chicken and mushrooms.

- 1 pound asparagus spears
- 2 cloves garlic, minced
- 20 black olives, pitted and halved
- 2 tablespoons olive oil
- ½ teaspoon salt
- ¼ teaspoon black pepper
- ½ cup water

Trim tough stems from asparagus and set aside.

Place a large skillet over medium heat and sauté garlic and olives in olive oil, 4 to 5 minutes.

Add asparagus, salt, pepper, and water.

Cover and cook over medium heat until asparagus is tender, 3 to 5 minutes.

Serve warm or cool.

Simple and Savory Scallop Salad

Hot salads make every meal look special. This favorite of ours came from one of our trips to the Great Barrier Reef. By the time we came back from our scuba dive, most of the buffet had been put away. A variation on this dish was all that remained but it was all that we needed to warm and nourish us.

2 tablespoons olive oil	2 ounces smoked salmon, cut into pieces
4 ounces sea scallops	
4 ounces mushrooms	4 large romaine lettuce leaves, washed
2 ounces fresh spinach, torn into pieces	

Heat olive oil over high heat. Add scallops and sauté for 2 minutes, until cooked thoroughly but not overdone. Remove to large bowl.

Add mushrooms, spinach, and smoked salmon and toss.

Serve over romaine lettuce leaves.

Tangy Steamed Cauliflower

*People don't always take the time to give vegetables an
opportunity to show off their good taste. Here's a quick-fix veggie
pleaser that we hope will make your friends sit up and take
notice.*

2   cups water
1   small cauliflower
4   tablespoons olive oil
2   tablespoons white vinegar
    salt to taste
    ground black pepper to
    taste

6   parsley sprigs, chopped
    fine
1/2 tablespoon grated
    Parmesan or Romano
    cheese
    hot sauce to taste

Place water in a saucepan and bring to a boil.

Wash cauliflower and cut into quarters, leaving green
leaves.

Add cauliflower quarters to boiling water, cover pan,
lower heat, and simmer 6 minutes.

Mix oil and vinegar in a bowl to make dressing; season
to taste.

Drain cauliflower, place in the bowl, and turn gently in
dressing until cauliflower is coated.

Sprinkle parsley over cauliflower.

Sprinkle with grated cheese.

Add hot sauce to taste, and serve at room temperature.

Skewered Fish

Timing is the key to the best skewered fish. Give the fish a full 5 minutes to marinate (10 minutes if possible) and stop cooking it when the fish is thoroughly done but not overcooked.

½ pound flounder fillets	1 green bell pepper, quartered
3 tablespoons olive oil	
juice of ½ lemon	4 large mushroom caps
2 green scallions, chopped	2 large romaine lettuce leaves, rinsed

Preheat broiler.

Cut fish into small squares and put into a bowl.

Pour olive oil and lemon juice over fish.

Add scallions to bowl and let fish marinate in mixture for 5 minutes.

Thread fish squares with alternate pieces of green pepper and mushroom caps on thin wooden skewers.

Place skewers on a baking sheet and broil for 5 to 10 minutes, until cooked thoroughly but not overdone. (Fish may also be cooked on an electric or outdoor grill.)

Baste fish 2 or 3 times while cooking, and turn skewers as fish colors.

Remove from skewers and place equal portions on lettuce leaves.

Serve immediately.

Low-Carb Mushroom Soup

Enjoy this dish as a soup or a sauce. Simply add less water and warm over low heat if you desire to make a nice, thick, tasty sauce for meat, poultry, or vegetables.

1 cup water	¼ cup heavy cream
1 pound mushrooms, cleaned and sliced	¼ cup grated Parmesan cheese
1 tablespoon olive oil	black pepper to taste

Bring water to boil in a sauté pan, add mushrooms, and boil slowly 4 to 5 minutes.

Drain and purée in a blender, adding olive oil and cream.

Empty into a bowl and stir in cheese and pepper to taste.

Poached Salmon Northwest

Portland, Oregon, and Seattle, Washington, have some of the finest seafood restaurants in the country. This dish was inspired by several of the best poached salmon recipes we were lucky enough to sample.

4	cups water	4	peppercorns
1	cup cauliflower florets	1	teaspoon lemon juice
1	celery stalk, diced	½	pound salmon fillet
1	bay leaf		

While heating water to boiling in a large saucepan, add cauliflower and celery into pan.

Add bay leaf, peppercorns, and lemon juice; boil slowly 5 minutes.

Reduce heat to simmer and add fish.

Gently simmer 5 minutes or until fish flakes when tested with a fork.

With a slotted spoon, remove salmon and cauliflower and place on a plate to cool.

Serve warm or cold.

Add celery, stir, and spoon over bed of watercress.

Green Pepper Salad with a Bite

Cool and hot, this is one of our good old dependables.

$^1/_2$ cup sour cream
1 teaspoon lemon juice
  dash Tabasco sauce
  salt to taste
  paprika to taste

2 cups diced green bell peppers
2 teaspoons chopped onions
6 fresh parsley sprigs, chopped

In a medium bowl, combine sour cream and lemon juice.
  Stir in Tabasco, salt, and paprika to taste.
  Stir green pepper and onions into bowl and mix well with sour cream sauce.
  Add parsley and serve.

Baked Flounder Italiano

Low-carb meals don't mean you have to give up Italian cooking. Add some mozzarella cheese as well for a special treat.

¼ cup olive oil	1 tablespoon dry white wine
½ pound flounder fillets	sea salt to taste
2 celery stalks, chopped	black pepper to taste
¼ cup grated Parmesan cheese	1 lemon, quartered

Preheat oven to 400°F.

Coat a baking dish with olive oil and lay in fillets. Place chopped celery around fillets.

Sprinkle cheese over fillets and celery.

Place dish in oven and bake for 5 minutes.

Drizzle wine into bottom of dish and baste fish; season to taste.

Return dish to oven, cook 5 to 6 minutes, and baste again.

Fish should flake when done.

Garnish with quartered lemon and serve.

Creamy Asian-Style Scallops

When we think about Asian cooking, we don't often think of cream sauces, but we love the way that the creaminess and Asian flavors work together in this dish.

2 tablespoons olive oil	paprika to taste
2 scallions, diced	1 teaspoon teriyaki sauce*
½ cup heavy cream	4 parsley sprigs, chopped
½ pound scallops	

Place olive oil in a sauté pan or skillet over medium heat.
Add scallions and stir until soft, about 1 minute.
Pour in cream, raise heat, and boil for 2 minutes.
Add scallops and cook slowly, 2 to 3 minutes.
Season with paprika, add teriyaki sauce, and cook 1 minute longer. Sprinkle with parsley and serve.

*Most recent Carbohydrate Addict's books may contain alternative guidelines for this ingredient. Consult your book's food lists for guidance. Use acceptable alternative as appropriate.

QUICK FIX DISHES AND SNACKS ❖ 277

Creamy Swiss Baked Eggs

This breakfast takes a minute to make but satisfies for hours.

1 tablespoon olive oil	1 cup sour cream
4 eggs	1 cup grated Swiss cheese

Preheat oven to 450°F.

Oil a medium-size baking dish. Beat eggs lightly, adding sour cream.

Pour egg mixture into baking dish; sprinkle with grated cheese.

Bake 10 minutes.

Tarragon Lamb Chops

SERVES 2

Faster than a frozen dinner and just as easy, but low-carb and delicious all the way.

2	large lamb chops, 1 inch thick	1	tablespoon dried tarragon salt to taste
4	tablespoons olive oil		black pepper to taste

Preheat broiler.

Place baking sheet in oven to heat.

Remove all fat from chops.

Combine olive oil, tarragon, salt, and pepper and coat both sides of each chop with the mixture.

Place chops on preheated baking sheet and broil for about 7 minutes; turn chops and broil for 5 minutes more.

Serve chops with remaining herby oil sprinkled on top of each chop.

Lemony Chicken Supreme

SERVES 4

We love to serve this dish to company and family who think we spent all day slaving over a hot stove.

1 egg yolk	2 tablespoons olive oil
¾ cup chicken stock, homemade only (page 26), or water	2 cups mushrooms
	salt to taste
	black pepper taste
3 tablespoons grated Parmesan cheese	½ lemon, cut in half
1 pound boneless, skinless chicken breasts, cut in 1-inch strips	

Beat egg yolk in a bowl with 2 tablespoons chicken stock (or water); stir in grated cheese.

Coat chicken strips with this egg batter. In a saucepan, heat olive oil, add chicken strips, and cook over medium heat until golden on all sides, about 4 minutes.

Remove chicken from pan to a warm dish; put mushrooms into pan over medium heat; add remaining stock, stirring to loosen all cooked bits from the bottom of pan.

Cook mushrooms about 5 minutes.

Season to taste. Combine chicken and mushrooms together on plates. Pour on sauce from pan and garnish with quartered lemon.

Hearty Asparagus with Eggs

We often enjoy this complete low-carb meal for a hearty breakfast or a quick and fun lunch.

2 tablespoons olive oil	4 eggs
8 asparagus spears, cut in 2-inch pieces	½ cup grated Cheddar cheese
4 slices beef sausage (no filler, no glutamates), cooked and drained	black pepper to taste

Preheat oven to 400°F.

Heat olive oil in a sauté pan or skillet.

Add asparagus pieces and cook for 2 minutes.

Place slices of cooked sausage on bottom of a medium-size ovenproof dish and add asparagus pieces. Break eggs into dish, and sprinkle ¼ cup cheese over eggs.

Pour pan juices over eggs and asparagus; sprinkle remaining ¼ cup grated cheese over all.

Bake for 4 to 5 minutes. Season to taste with pepper.

Rainbow Casserole

We first made this dish from leftovers in an iron skillet over a campfire at Walt Disney World Campground. The fragrance of this casserole takes us back to those wonderful memories every time.

2 slices bacon*	1 pound green beans, trimmed
8 ounces sliced leftover pork	
2 cups chopped cauliflower	½ cup water

In a small skillet, fry the bacon strips.

Pour off excess grease, but leave enough to coat bottom of pan.

Add sliced pork.

Add cauliflower, green beans, and water.

Cover and cook until cauliflower and green beans are done, approximately 7 minutes.

Serve warm.

*Most recent Carbohydrate Addict's books may contain alternative guidelines for this ingredient. Consult your book's food lists for guidance. Use acceptable alternative as appropriate.

Everything Omelette

We call this our "pile it on, eat it up" omelette. It's different every time we make it, and that's part of its charm. Substitute your low-carb leftovers for ours in this recipe.

4	large eggs	4	ounces cooked pork
1	teaspoon water	½	cup grated Cheddar cheese
	salt to taste		
	black pepper to taste	2	celery stalks, diced
1	tablespoon olive oil	1	green bell pepper, diced

In a medium bowl, combine eggs, water, salt, and pepper.

Heat the olive oil in a skillet over medium heat and add the egg mixture. Use a small spatula run around the edges of the skillet to free the edges.

Tip the skillet so the uncooked egg from the center of the pan can run under the bottom of the cooked egg.

Continue to do this until the egg in the center is still just a little moist. Add pork, cheese, celery, and green pepper chunks to omelet as desired.

Roll the omelet with three folds as you turn it onto a serving plate. Divide into two equal portions and serve immediately.

Spinach Omelet with Sour Cream

SERVES 2

This dish is easy enough to make in a few minutes but elegant enough to serve to guests.

4   large eggs
1   teaspoon water
    salt to taste
    black pepper to taste
1   tablespoon olive oil

1   cup frozen spinach, thawed
4   tablespoons sour cream
1/2 teaspoon ground nutmeg

In a large bowl, combine eggs, water, salt, and pepper.

Heat olive oil in a skillet over medium heat and add the egg mixture.

Cook until the eggs are cooked thoroughly but are not rubbery.

Sprinkle the spinach in and top it with sour cream; sprinkle with nutmeg, then roll the omelet with three folds as you turn it onto a serving plate.

Divide into two equal portions and serve immediately.

Index

A Final Note Until We See You Again

WE HAD A WONDERFUL TIME PREPARING THESE RECIPES. As we cooked up each dish, you were always on our minds. We wanted you to discover a world of exciting, fun, and easy delights and to celebrate the joy of eating without guilt.

We hope that you will return to these pages again and again and that some of our favorites will become yours as well. Good friends, good food, and the time to enjoy them both: these are the blessings of a good life.

With our warmest wishes,

Drs. Richard and Rachael Heller